Endomorph Diet

*Burn Fat According to Your Body Type with
Keto Diet, Intermittent Fasting and Exercises
to Dramatically Improve Your Body Shape for
The Rest of Your Life*

Emma Moore

Table of Contents

INTRODUCTION

The diet for endomorph not only aims to lose weight, but also focuses on reducing fat mass to reach less than 25% of total fat mass in women and less than 20% in men. When the above goals are achieved, you can start working simultaneously to gain muscle. Slow metabolism results in lower daily caloric expenditure . Then, if an endomorphic person consumes a few extra calories, this will quickly translate into an increase in weight. And the same happens with carbohydrates, which are quickly transformed into adipose tissue (fat). The total caloric value of the diet will depend on weight, height, sex and physical activity, among other factors. However, it is not advisable to obsess over calories, but pay attention to the quality of the food and the size of the portions. The daily distribution of macronutrients that diets for endomorphs should have to burn fat and lose weight should be 25% carbohydrates, 35% protein and 40% fat. Perhaps some people might think that the feeding of an endomorph to lose fat should be low fat (less than 20% fat) but this is not true, since monounsaturated fats (such as olive oil or avocado) and polyunsaturated fats (such as fish, nuts and seeds) contribute to weight loss, reduce inflammation, normalize cholesterol levels and prevent the formation of atheromatous plaques so frequent in people with this somatotype. Carbohydrates are reduced because endomorphs tend to have insulin resistance.It is recommended that they be whole carbohydrates, avoiding refined foods that raise blood sugar levels abruptly and, consequently, those of insulin.Carbohydrates should be reserved for pre-workout and post-workout snacks.Proteins are the key nutrients to lose weight because they increase metabolic expenditure by thermogenesis associated with food, in addition to providing a lot of satiety. The endomorphic people are characterized by having a rounded body, because of its ability to accumulate fat. It is not surprising that individuals who belong to this biotype are overweight or obese because of their slow metabolism. In order to maintain weight and fat mass within normal parameters, they must perform cardiovascular physical activity routines and have a healthy diet. However, contrary to what is usually believed, endomorphs do not have a hard time increasing their muscle mass and obtain excellent results with anaerobic training.

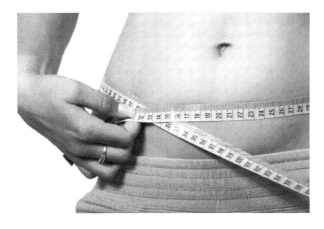

CHAPTER ONE:
What Exactly Is An Endomorph

In the area of health, science and sports it is considered that all people, from the moment they are born, belong to one of the three types of body structure that exist and that have been studied: mesomorph, ectomorph or endomorph . The physical characteristics of people and their sporting achievements will always depend on these types of texture. However, thanks to the training that has been created over time and proper nutrition, it is now possible to change the "own" somatotype and move from being a very thin build to an entire athlete. However, these aspects also depend on the tendencies granted by nature and genetics. The endomorph body type stores more fat than average, gets tired easily, and has a larger appetite, making it difficult to lose weight. Their build is wider than an ectomorph or mesomorph, with a larger bone structure, more strength, and accompanied by significantly more body fat.

We could define an endomorph (male or female) as someone who shares with the ectomorphs the difficulties to gain muscle, but it differs from them by its great ease to gain fat. That's right, the worst of both worlds . They are also typically distinguished by certain anatomical qualities: short extremities, wider hips (same height as the shoulders or more) and generally rounder shapes. In addition, they usually have wider joints. Quick test: surround your left wrist with the thumb and middle finger of the right hand. If both fingers do not touch, you have wide joints.

Beyond the external appearance, the endomorphs usually share some physiological characteristics:

- Slower metabolism . Genetics impacts on our basal metabolism, or the calories we burn at rest. But also in caloric partitioning, or in other words, in what happens with the calories consumed. The hormonal environment and other physiological aspects of endomorphs tend to accumulate more calories as fat and less as muscle.
- Lower caloric expenditure through thermogenesis not associated with exercise, which some experts associate to which of our nervous systems predominates: the sympathetic ('fight and flight) in the ectomorphs or the parasympathetic (' rest and digestion ') in the endomorphs.
- Greater number of fat cells and / or greater sensitivity to insulin in fat cells .
- Less muscle fibers and / or less sensitivity to insulin in muscle tissue .

Types Of Bodies: Ectomorph, Mesomorph Or Endomorph.

It is very important to be able to identify and understand what our body type is. In this article we will learn to differentiate the three different types of structure: ectomorph, mesomorph and endomorph, together with their physical characteristics.

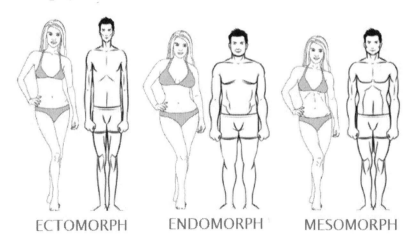

ECTOMORPH   ENDOMORPH   MESOMORPH

Body Type: Ectomorph

An ectomorph is the typical thin person. In general, the typical ectomorph has long, thin legs with very fibrous muscles. The shoulders tend to be thin with little width.

Typical features of an ectomorph

- Thin build Of thin bone
- Flat chest
- Small shoulders

- Lean muscle mass
- Does not gain weight easily
- Rapid metabolism

Type of training:

Brief and high intensity
Focusing the workout on large muscle groups
Ectomorphs find it very difficult to gain weight. They have a metabolism so fast that it burns calories quickly. As a general rule, they need a large amount of calories in order to gain weight.

Workouts should be short and intense, focusing on large muscle groups.Ectomorphs should eat before going to bed to avoid muscle catabolism at night.In general, gaining muscle is a somewhat complex task for this type of body.

Body type: Mesomorph

A mesomorph has a large bone structure, strong muscles and a natural athlete physique. Mesomorphs are the best body type for bodybuilding and a lot of sports. They find it very easy to gain and lose weight. They are strong by nature, which is the perfect platform for building muscle.

Typical features in a mesomorph

- Wide shoulders
- Athletic
- Strong body with defined muscles
- Rectangular shaped body
- They gain muscles easily

- They gain fat with some ease

The mesomorphic body type responds better to weight training.The gains are usually seen very quickly, especially in the beginners.The disadvantage is that mesomorphs gain fat more easily than ectomorphs. This means that they must monitor their calorie intake or they will gain weight quickly. In general, a combination of weight training and cardio works best for mesomorphs

Training Type:

Cardio routines
Various weight routines
Control calorie consumption

Body Type: Endomorph
The endomorphic body type is usually soft and flaccid. Endomorphs gain fat very easily. Endomorphs tend to have thin arms and broad legs. The muscles are strong and powerful, especially those of the legs.Endomorphs are naturally strong in leg exercises like the squat.
Typical features of an endomorph
- Soft round shape
- Gain muscle and fat easily
- Slow metabolism
- Giant and chunky physicist
- It's hard to lose fat
- Your slow metabolism
- It's hard to define your muscles

Type Of Training:

Cardiac routines + Weight management for toning

Controlling calorie consumption

When it comes to training for endomorphs, they find it very easy to gain weight. Unfortunately, a large part of this weight is fat, not muscle. To encourage muscle gain compared to fat, you should perform aerobic activities.They assimilate proteins very well, so they do not need to supplement.

CHAPTER TWO:
Why It's Hard To Watch Your Weight As An Endomorph

Why is it so horribly difficult for people like me to lose weight fast and keep it off?

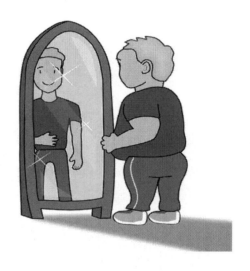

I am an endomorph. I am a pear shaped endomorph who hangs onto every shred of fat by my hips and thighs.

It could be worse. I could be an apple shaped endomorph and if you are reading this and thinking "Hang on, that's me. What's she on about?" the answer is potentially quite a lot.

You apple shaped girls and guys have your fat storage around your upper body and that's where your heart and lungs need some breathing space to keep you alive. Fat around the top is dangerous fat, so it's got to come off or it will keep applying more and more discomforting and dangerous pressure to these vital organs.

It's just not fair. My husband is a mesomorph and he can eat much more than me, exercise less rigorously and maintain the weight he wants with ease. Now that's partly because men carry less fat anyway and they also burn more calories by nature, but it also has a lot to do with the forgiving nature of the mesomorph body compared to the grudging nature of the endomorph frame.

Whether we resemble an apple or a pear, diet and exercise is a real struggle for us endomorphs compared to the 2 other body shapes our parents could have bequeathed us.

The up and down ectomorph can eat anything but they do get a bit of a flabby tummy effect if they eat badly, which they often do. The superior mesomorph (hourglass shaped women and wide shouldered, slim hipped men) can drop weight and get moving fast and furiously with zest and determination for however long it takes to reach their goal.

We endomorphs are different. For us to lose weight fast we need a really strict and clean diet (with one or two cheat meals a week to keep us from going mean and snappy) and a regular exercise program, mainly cardio, 5-6 sessions a week.

We are by nature more slothlike than either the ectomorph (whose nervous energy burns calories standing still) or the mesomorph (whose strength and determination will see them achieve ANYTHING they want to). We tend not to push ourselves until we have a REALLY good reason to do so. And we are excellent at talking ourselves out of clean diet and regular exercise.

To lose weight fast, the humble endomorph have to hone in on some tricks for our body type. We have to latch onto a motivation, a compelling and highly personal reason to lose weight fast. Once we have the reason, we can turn our weight loss dreams into reality.

Yes, it surely is more difficult for us to lose weight fast, but with the right mindset it definitely can be done.

The Right Mindset

It is obvious that before eating your food you buy it, your responsibility is to choose the healthy ones. So it is always the most appropriate time of the year to clean up your food shelves and throw away foods that will just make you fat. Grat part of your decision to lose body fat is to lose those nasty food cravings that are far from healthy. Be sure to dispose of foods that are rich in sugar and unhealthy fat.

After cleaning your food cabinets off bad food, put in healthy ones such as whole grains, fruits and veggies and other high-fiber foods. It is also important that you consume foods that are rich in protein namely white meat, beans, and nuts. You are able to surely cook up a meal strategy which will ensure that you are receiving the adequate amount of nutrients that your entire body requires for it to become functioning well. Learning how to lose body fat the healthy way through healthy way is like the greatest favor you can give to your body.

Make sure to improve fluid intake. Water is recognized to remove harmful toxins and deposits of extra fat in the body, so drinking 8 to 10 glasses of water daily, together with your high-fiber diet plan will aid you eliminate your fat quickly.

How to eradicate body fat? Participate in a holistic weight training.

It would be really great if you can maintain a regular workout schedule that fits your fitness level. Choose a workout routine that will strengthen various muscle groups. A holistic body workout is essential in decreasing your body fat percentage. Always make sure that your workout plan matches that of your bodily requirements. In case things are not very clear to you yet, ask the assistance of a fitness instructor to help you understand your situation better.

For you to have a good start in working out, try aerobics or a dance fitness class. There are those who instantly find lifting weights and counting reps extremely boring. It is sad that oftentimes, boredom just gets in the way of having a beautiful body. Thankfully, cardio and aerobics sessions tend to be more alive and enjoyable because it is more of a social event. Moreover, there's some dance music to set you into the groove. Those who find it hard to work out might find the answer in this particular form of exercise.

CHAPTER THREE:
How To Lose Weight With The Ketogenic Diet

Weight Loss Issues for Endomorph Body Types

An endomorph body type is often characterized by fuller figures. Most endomorphs also complain that they have a difficult time maintaining a healthy body fat percentage. It is mainly because of their tendency to gain weight easily.With that in mind, it is no longer surprising to see endomorphs struggling with their weight.They often find it hard to lose weight and find the perfect diet plan for them. However, by understanding the common weight loss issues that plague endomorphs, finding the most appropriate diet plan for you will be much easier. Here are the most common issues associated with losing weight that you might encounter if you are an endomorph.

Slow or poor metabolism – As an endomorph, you will most likely have a poor or slower metabolism. Naturally, you will have a sluggish metabolic rate. There is no need to worry too much, though, as this does not necessarily mean that you are going to be obese or overweight forever. Just making some changes in the foods you eat can help in firing up your metabolic rate.

Gains weight easily – As mentioned earlier, endomorphs are prone to gaining weight fast. The weight that you will most likely accumulate will usually be on your hips, thighs, and low belly. You also tend to store fat. Again, the best way to handle this is to eat the right foods. Combine it with proper exercise, too.

Sensitivity to extra calories – One major reason why endomorphs tend to struggle more when it comes to their weight than the other different body types, like ectomorph and mesomorph, is their sensitivity to excessive food consumption.In other words, burning calories is a bit hard for you. In fact, you will most likely store extra calories as fat, causing you to accumulate weight.

Sensitivity to carbs and insulin – Another issue associated with weight loss that you will most likely encounter as an endomorph is your sensitivity to carbs and insulin. Because you are carb-sensitive, you will have a higher chance of surviving better and losing weight if you follow a low-carb diet.

While being an endomorph causes you to encounter a few weight loss challenges, it does not mean that you can't lose weight or maintain a healthy and fit figure. All it takes is to adhere to the healthiest eating and exercise plan.

Ideal Endomorph Diet Approach

The ideal diet plan for endomorphs is actually a low-carb diet. In this case, you should develop your diet plan in such a way that your fat and protein intake will be higher when compared to carbs. Your carb intake should be brought down to the minimum. The perfect macronutrient ratio for you, therefore, is 30 to 40% carbs, 30 to 35% protein, and 30 to 35% fat. As a start, you may have more carbs when distributing the nutrients. For instance, you can set your diet plan at 40% carbs then 30% each of healthy fats and proteins. However, if you still notice that you don't lose weight, then you can further decrease your carb consumption and distribute the remaining percentage equally between protein and fats. The goal of any your endomorph diet is to stay away from starchy carbs and white bread. You also have to incorporate healthy fats into your diet plan, such as olive oil, which is a good source of it.You don't need to make everything too complicated, though.The ratio of fat, carbs, and protein does not even have to be exactly accurate.

Protein: The Key to Endomorph Weight Loss

In general, it just involves developing a diet plan composed of foods that are higher in fat and lean protein and lower in carbohydrates.What's good about the low-carb diet is that it can help endomorphs in losing excess fats while maintaining their energy levels. The higher protein consumption also promotes a lower calorie intake without making you feel hungry and deprived. It is mainly because a meal rich in protein is known to be more satisfying. It can make you feel fuller compared to when you are eating a carb-heavy meal. Your lower carb intake combined with higher amounts of protein can also prevent you from losing muscles, which usually happens once you lower calories for weight loss.The low-carb diet is also good for endomorphs as this can supply them with just the right amount of carbs to serve as fuel for their metabolic needs while controlling their blood sugar.

What are ketone bodies?
The name ketogenic diet means, in reality, that it creates ketone bodies. Ketone bodies are a metabolic product that is generated when the body does not have available carbohydrates to burn quickly. Therefore, this diet rejects carbohydrates to the maximum, using fat as an energy source and increasing the amount of protein. Let's take a quick look at what happens in our body when we need energy. Imagine the muscle as a powerful machine that needs fuel.The fastest and most immediate fuel is the concentration of glucose in the blood. If our blood glucose is very low and energy expenditure increases, the muscle soon loses its sustenance. Then it will take advantage of another store of stored carbohydrates: glycogen. If the body also remains without this reserve, then, it will return to another metabolic pathway: ketosis .Ketosis occurs mainly in the liver, where the fat will transform, after a short journey, into ketone bodies. Normally, fat is used to produce energy through the Krebs cycle. However, in desperate situations, some components of the fatty acids go to a faster but less efficient metabolism.
It produces "special" molecules (such as acetoacetyl coenzyme A) that end up giving acetone, acetoacetic acid or

beta-hydroxybutyric acid.Or, in other words, ketone bodies. Ketone bodies are used with the immediacy of glucose, to obtain energy, at the expense of fats, which will help us explain some of the evidence we will discuss.

Why does the ketogenic diet work?

Ketogenic diets have been shown in several studies to be effective when losing weight.This is based on three facts. The first, of which we spoke before, is that this diet takes advantage of fats quickly, using a more inefficient route. Inefficient, in this case, suits us because it indicates that we need more fat for the production of less energy

The second is that it prevents hypercaloric intake and the accumulation of fats due to excess carbohydrates. Normal diets contain a large amount of carbohydrates (a large amount does not imply too many, it all depends on the diet). With a ketogenic diet, it is impossible to accumulate an excess of glucose in the blood and, therefore, of fat coming from an excess of energy.

The third, according to some studies, is that the ketogenic diet helps to maintain satiety levels, helping to better control the intake in patients who practice it.Following this trio of effects, studies have proven that it can be useful to reduce obesity.

When and how should we use it?

The ketogenic diet should be used as a tool for certain circumstances. It must be made clear that the exclusionary approach of this type of diet does not match the idea of healthy habits.A balanced and healthy diet includes legumes, cereals, fruits ... a series of foods that can be rich in carbohydrates.Ketogenic pattern diets, however, bypass these macronutrients to induce ketosis.

This can be useful for weight control, as we said, in patients with obesity. They can also help us if we plan them with a specialist so that we avoid the problems we mentioned. Another use of the ketogenic diet is to use it in the last stage of muscle definition.

In this case, it is convenient to combine it with a hyper-prosthetic diet to avoid the loss of muscle mass and maximize its growth. Finally, maintaining a state of permanent ketosis is not very advisable, although well taken does not have to be a problem. But always with strict control.

How to Start a Ketogenic Diet for Weight Loss

A ketogenic diet (also known as "nutritional ketosis") is a high-fat, adequate-protein, low-carbohydrate diet. On a ketogenic diet, your brain uses ketones (a byproduct of your fat-burning metabolism) for fuel, instead of glucose. Since humans can burn either glucose or ketones for energy, this change is possible to make, although there is some controversy surrounding ketogenic diets regarding both their efficacy and health benefit.

Ketosis keeps your body in a "fasting" or starvation metabolism, and consequently encourages weight loss by burning off fat reserves. While the shift to a ketogenic diet can be difficult initially, you should begin to see results after a few weeks.

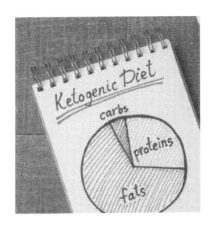

1. Beginning a Ketogenic Diet

Talk to your doctor. Although the ketogenic diet is grounded in medical and nutritional fact, there is not a universal opinion in the medical community that the diet is effective for weight-loss. Your personal doctor will be able to advise you if the diet is a good fit for you personally.

- Some sources view a ketogenic diet as an effective way to counter the symptoms of certain illnesses — such as epilepsy — rather than a weight-loss diet.
- If you are pregnant or diabetic, work with your doctor so they can monitor and adjust your medications while you follow this diet.
- If you are type-1 diabetic, seek permission from a doctor well-trained in nutrition before you start this diet.

Recognize the possible risks of a ketogenic diet. A ketogenic diet — and putting your body into ketosis generally — presents risks for anyone who suffers from heart or kidney problems.If you are at risk for heart disease or kidney disease, avoid ketogenic diets.

- A ketogenic diet prescribes moderate amounts of proteins, and large amounts of fats.
- A ketogenic diet will also add strain to your kidneys. Protein-heavy foods increase the amount of calcium in your urine. This, in turn, can strain your kidneys and lead to the development of kidney stones.

Start with a general low-carb diet like Atkins to ease yourself into nutritional ketosis. The Atkins diet is heavy on fats and proteins, low on carbohydrates, and will encourage your body to burn ketones for energy. Atkins is a decent "middle ground" between a regular diet (often high in carbs) and a low-protein ketogenic diet.

- This step is optional, but may make the transitional period into a ketogenic diet easier.

Calculate your "macronutrients."

Macronutrients are nutrients which your body needs in large quantities, and they provide energy in the form of calories. Calculating your macronutrient intake will let you see the current levels of your fat consumption. With this information, you can decide how to reduce your carb and protein consumption, and increase your fat consumption.

- There are three types of macronutrients: fats, proteins, and carbohydrates. Fats provide more calories per gram than either proteins or carbs.

- There are many macronutrient calculators available online. You'll need to input your height, weight, daily exercise, and dietary information

2. Adjusting your Diet

Eat as much as 20 or 30 grams of carbs daily. If you determine — through a macronutrient calculator — that you currently eat more than 30 grams of carbs daily, look for ways to decrease your carb intake. It's crucial to avoid carbs on a ketogenic diet, as carbs easily convert into glucose, which keeps your body from burning ketones for energy.

- You should only receive about 5–10% of your daily calories from carbohydrates, by eating about 20 – 30 grams a day.
- Focus on getting your carbs through salad greens and non-starchy vegetables only.
- Avoid carb-heavy foods like pasta and bread.

Eat 2 – 8 ounces of protein several times a day. Protein is a necessary part of your diet, and without proteins, you will have very little energy. You may also feel hungrier or develop food cravings throughout the day.However, too much protein will diminish the weight-loss effects of a ketogenic diet.

- You should aim to consume about 25 – 30% of your daily calories from proteins.
- The amount of protein you eat will vary depending on how much protein you require as an individual. This is often tied to lifestyle, whether active or sedentary.

Eat fats with all your meals. Fats are the cornerstone of the ketogenic diet, and will encourage your body to burn fatty ketones for fuel. Typically, calories from fat should comprise 80 – 90% of your meals.(However, you cannot eat unlimited fats on a ketogenic diet; the calories can still add up and cause weight gain. Examples of fatty foods include:

- Organic butter and lard
- Coconut oil
- Fatty cuts of organic, grass-fed meat.
- Egg yolks and full-fat sour cream
- Homemade mayonnaise
- Heavy whipping cream and cream cheese
- Avocados and bacon
- Nuts and nut butters

Don't stress too much about calories. Unlike many other weight-loss diets, you do not need to actively keep track of the number of calories in the dishes you eat while on a ketogenic diet. Since a ketogenic diet reduces food cravings throughout the day, you'll likely be less motivated to eat excess calories anyway.

- If you do want to track your calories, use the following breakdown as a guide (assuming that you'll consume about 1,500 calories a day):
- 1,050 calories from fat
- 300 calories from protein
- 150 calories from carbohydrates

Stay hydrated. Once your body is in ketosis, your kidneys will begin to release excess water which your body had been retaining. This retained water is a consequence of a high-carb diet, and once you reduce your carb intake, water retention will decrease as well.

- As a consequence, you may need to increase your daily water intake to avoid dehydration.
- Headaches and muscle cramps are a sign of dehydration. You may also need to increase mineral intake, especially salt and magnesium, as these are often lost when your body gets rid of retained water.

3. Losing Weight on Your Diet

Use a ketone meter to test whether you are in ketosis. A ketone meter will measure a small sample of your blood, calculate your blood sugar, and will inform you if your body is in ketosis.

- Certain ketone meters test urine rather than blood; however, testing your blood is more accurate than testing your urine.
- Ketone meters are commonly for sale at drug stores, and also online.
- If you are in ketosis, your body will burn its fat reserves, and you will begin to notice weight loss.

Look for ketosis symptoms (also known as "keto flu"). Within three to seven days of starting the diet, you may notice symptoms like: strong-smelling breath or urine; slight nausea; high energy and mental clarity; fatigue; or diminished appetite with no cravings.

- If these symptoms last longer than a week, or increase in severity, you should visit your doctor. Severe nausea can lead to vomiting and dehydration, which are unhealthy when continued for multiple days.
- Many of these symptoms will vanish once you become keto-adapted.
- This symptom analysis can be performed in place of testing, if you are limited financially or do not want to test your blood or urine.

Notice that your health has improved (after a few weeks). This should also be accompanied by weight loss, and any bloating or inflammation which you had previously experienced will have improved greatly.

- Ketogenic recipes are readily available online. Search online for various keto-friendly sites.
- Search in Pinterest (or similar apps) for good ketogenic recipes.
- Common recipes include rich "fat bomb" desserts, low-carb sandwiches, and light meals with avocado and salmon

14 Days Endomorph Diet Plan

Cook one, two or three times a day

Here are 42 recipes for breakfast, lunch and dinner for each day for two weeks, ideal if you like to vary. But if you want to cook less, you can do two things:

Simplify lunch: cook two servings at dinner and refrigerate the second to serve lunch the next day. Voilà : there is no need to prepare lunch!

Simplify breakfast: You could choose one of the keto breakfasts you like and repeat it every day; like the scrambled eggs .Or, if you're not hungry, you can skip breakfast and maybe just have a coffee.This not only saves you time and money, it also increases the concentration of ketones in your blood.

Get ready

A ketogenic diet is suitable for most people, but in the following situations you may need additional support:

Checklist

Are you taking medications for diabetes, eg insulin?

Are you taking medication for hypertension?

Are you breastfeeding?

If none of these cases apply to you, you are ready to begin.

Just remember one last thing if you are just starting to eat keto: you need to drink enough fluids and increase your salt intake during the first week to avoid the flu ketone and feel the best you can. For example, taking a cup of broth 1-2 times a day helps a lot.

Let's continue to the ketogenic menu for 14 days.

DAY ONE

BREAKFAST
(SCRAMBLED EGGS)

Butter + eggs = the perfect ketogenic breakfast. This is how the day begins, with a particularly delicious and buttery version of this classic breakfast. And it's ready in just a few minutes!

INGREDIENTS
- 2 eggs
- 30 g butter
- Salt and ground black pepper

INSTRUCTIONS
- Beat the eggs together with some salt and pepper using a fork.
- Melt the butter in a nonstick skillet over medium heat. Look closely: butter does not turn golden!
- Pour the eggs into the pan and mix for 1-2 minutes until they are creamy and cooked a little less than you like. Remember that the eggs will continue to cook even once you put them on your plate.

TIPS!

These creamy eggs pair well with many popular low carb dishes. Of course, there is the option of eating them with classic accompaniments such as bacon or sausage, but there are other great options such as salmon, avocado, cold cuts and cheese (cheddar, fresh mozzarella or feta).

And if you're very hungry (or are cooking with large eggs), do not be shy: use more butter!

LUNCH
(COLD CUTS OF ROAST BEEF WITH COLESLAW)

Let's drink by not cooking tonight. Using good quality grilled meat meats means that you can enjoy a tasty and nutritious meal without a lot of work in the kitchen. It is a substantial keto meal that you can prepare very quickly.

INGREDIENTS

- 300 ml (275 g) mayonnaise
- 1 tbsp Dijon mustard
- 450 g green cabbage
- 650 g meats of beef
- 110 g cherry tomatoes
- 4 pickles pickled with dill
- Salt and ground black pepper

INSTRUCTIONS

- Mix the mayonnaise and mustard in a large bowl. Salt and pepper to taste.

34

- Cut the cabbage into thin strips and add it to the bowl. Stir with the mayonnaise mixture and let stand for a couple of minutes.
- Place the roast beef, tomatoes and pickled cucumbers on a plate along with a good portion of coleslaw. Serve cold or at room temperature.

ADVICE!

Make it even easier by buying already cut cabbage! Just look at the nutrition information label to see if there are hidden carbohydrates (for example if mixed with other vegetables such as carrots). We do not recommend the cabbage salad that is bought in the supermarket or the deli: there is usually sugar in the dressing.

DINNER
(KETOGENIC PORK CHOPS WITH CABBAGE CASSEROLE)

Try this delicious cabbage casserole with a juicy pork chop and a good dose of parmesan butter melted on top. It's a great keto meal !

INGREDIENTS
- Cabbage casserole
- 900 g green cabbage
- 1 yellow onion
- 2 cloves of garlic
- 75 g butter

- 300 ml whipping cream
- 125 ml sour cream or fresh cream
- 150 g (150 ml) cream cheese
- 1 tbsp mix of ranch spices
- 1 tsp Salt
- ¼ tsp. ground black pepper
- 150 g grated cheese

Pork chops

- 6 pork chops
- Salt and ground black pepper
- 30 g butter

Parmesan butter

- 150 g butter
- 60 g parmesan cheese
- ½ tsp. sea salt
- 1 pinch ground black pepper

INSTRUCTIONS

- Remove butter and chops from the refrigerator and set aside at room temperature for later use.
- Preheat the oven to 200 ° C (400 ° F). Cut the onion, garlic and green cabbage into strips with a sharp knife, a mandolin slicer or in a food processor.
- Heat a large skillet and add butter. Sauté the vegetables for 10 minutes until they become soft but not browned.
- Add thick cream, sour cream, cream cheese and spices. Mix well and let simmer for another 5-10 minutes.

- Pour into a roasting pan. Sprinkle the cheese on top and bake for 20 minutes.
- Mix all the ingredients for the parmesan butter with a fork in a small bowl.
- Meanwhile, season the pork chops and fry them or grill them until they are fully cooked.
- Let the meat rest for a few minutes before serving with the casserole and parmesan butter.

ADVICE!

Another even simpler option is to use a couple of slices of roast beef, pastrami or a good quality sausage.

DAY TWO

BREAKFAST
(Ketogenic Frittata Of Goat Cheese And Mushrooms)

This tasty frittata with mushrooms, spinach and goat cheese gives you a keto and vegetarian meal that is quick to make and that really satisfies you.

INGREDIENTS
Frittata
- 150 g mushrooms
- 75 g fresh spinach
- 50 g chives
- 50 g butter
- 6 eggs
- 110 g goat cheese
- Salt and ground black pepper

At your service
- 150 g green leafy vegetables
- 2 tbsp olive oil
- Salt and ground black pepper

INSTRUCTIONS
- Preheat the oven to 175 ° C (350 ° F).
- Grate or crumble the cheese and mix in a bowl with the eggs. Salt and pepper to taste.

- Cut the mushrooms into small pieces. Chop the chives.
- Melt the butter over medium heat in a pan suitable for the oven and fry the mushrooms and onions for 5-10 minutes or until golden brown.
- Add the spinach to the pan and fry for another 1-2 minutes. Pepper.
- Pour the egg mixture in the pan. Bake for about 20 minutes or until browned and firm in the middle.

LUNCH
(CHICKEN AND BACON SALAD)

All these flavors together taste great: chicken, bacon, lettuce, tomato ... It's a great combination, but why leave it there? Make this delicious salad even more keto by adding a good dose of creamy alioli. Yes now!

INGREDIENTS
- 450 g boneless chicken thighs
- 30 g butter
- 225 g bacon
- 110 g cherry tomatoes
- 275 g romaine lettuce
- Salt and ground black pepper

Aioli
- 175 ml (150 g) mayonnaise
- ½ cda. garlic powder

INSTRUCTIONS

- Mix the mayonnaise and garlic powder in a small bowl and set aside.
- Fry the slices of bacon in butter until crispy. Remove them from the pan and keep them warm. Save the accumulated fat in the pan.
- Crumble the chicken and season it. Fry in the same pan as the chicken until golden brown and completely cooked.
- Rinse the lettuce and cut it into strips. Make sure you use a different cutting board than the one you used for the chicken. Put the lettuce on a plate with the chicken, bacon, tomatoes and a good dose of mayonnaise with garlic.

DINNER
(Thai Keto Curry With Fish And Coconut)

This is an easy way to cook fish with a lot of flavor. Perfect for those seeking ketogenic fast food and Asian flavors.

INGREDIENTS

- 30 g butter or olive oil, to grease the asadera
- 700 g salmon or white fish

- salt or ground black pepper
- 4 tbsp butter or ghee
- 2 tbsp red curry paste or green curry paste
- 400 g coconut cream
- 120 ml (8 g) fresh cilantro, chopped
- 450 g (1 liter) cauliflower or broccoli

INSTRUCTIONS

- Preheat the oven to 200 ° C (400 ° F). Grease a roasting pan.
- Put the pieces of fish in a medium roasting pan. There should not be much space between the edges of the broiler pan and the fish.
- Salt and pepper to taste. Put a spoonful of butter on each piece of fish.
- Mix the coconut cream, curry paste and chopped coriander in a small bowl and spread the mixture over the fish.
- Bake for 20 minutes or until the fish is ready.
- Boil the cauliflower or broccoli in slightly salted water for a couple of minutes and serve with the fish.

ADVICE

If you do not find coconut cream in the supermarket you can use coconut milk. In this case, use two cans and let them sit in the refrigerator for a few hours or overnight. Open the cans carefully and remove the coconut water. Do not bounce the water: you can use it in smoothies and other refreshing drinks.

DAY THREE

BREAKFAST
(Breakfast Caps)

If you are looking for a delicious dish to serve several people, look no further! If you use cheese, cold meats and nuts of good quality, you will have an exquisite ketogenic banquet in a very short time, and it is fresh, colorful and tasty.

INGREDIENTS
- An assortment of cheeses (for example mozzarella, cheddar, gouda and parmesan
- An assortment of cold meats (ham, raw ham, chorizo and salami)
- Cucumbers, peppers, radishes, pickles
- Avocado with homemade mayonnaise and pepper
- Nuts eg nuts, almonds or hazelnuts (low-carbohydrate nuts guide)
- fresh basil

INSTRUCTIONS
- Cut the cold meats, cheese and vegetables into sticks or cubes.
- Split the avocado and cut it into small slices.
- Mix with 100 g of homemade mayonnaise, 1 tablespoon of crushed grains of pink pepper and perhaps a bit of freshly squeezed lemon juice.

- Place the mixture in the avocado peels and serve.

ADVICE!
Do not wait until you have guests at home! This ingenious dish is so easy and fast that you can enjoy it at any time.

NOTE
This recipe does not carry nutritional information because we do not indicate the exact amounts of each ingredient. The exact figures will depend on how much you eat of each food!

LUNCH
(Keto Salmon With Broccoli And Lemon Mayonnaise)

This is another super simple dish that is perfect for someone who follows a strict ketogenic diet and wants something quick and tasty. Salmon and broccoli are fried in butter in the same pan: enjoy this mix of flavors with fresh lemon mayonnaise!

INGREDIENTS
- 225 ml (200 g) mayonnaise
- 2 tbsp lemon juice
- 650 g salmon
- 50 g butter
- 450 g broccoli
- Salt and ground black pepper

INSTRUCTIONS

- Mix mayonnaise and lemon juice. Salt and pepper to taste. Put aside.
- Fry the portions of salmon in half the butter over medium heat for a couple of minutes on each side. Lower the fire towards the end. Remove them from the pan and keep them warm.
- Rinse, dry and trim unusable parts of broccoli, including the stem. Chop into small pieces.
- Add the rest of the butter to the same pan you used for the salmon. Fry the broccoli over medium heat for 3-4 minutes, or until golden brown and soft. Salt and pepper to taste.
- Serve salmon and broccoli with a good dose of lemon mayonnaise.

DINNER
(Crispy Chicken Legs With Cole Slaw)

Let's raise the temperature! This chicken has a crispy, Jamaican-style crispy top with a spicy mix of spices. The recipe is perfect for legs or chicken wings. It's incredibly delicious and infinitely healthier than any equivalent in a restaurant or on the street.The same goes for coleslaw. So enjoy this ketogenic delight !

INGREDIENTS

- 900 g chicken legs

- 120 ml sour cream or Greek yogurt
- 2 tbsp olive oil
- 2 tbsp Jamaican-style spice mix
- 1 tsp Salt
- 150 g pork rinds
- 90 g grated coconut without sugar
- 60 ml olive oil

Cabbage salad
- 450 g green cabbage
- 240 ml (225 g) mayonnaise
- Salt and ground black pepper

INSTRUCTIONS
- Preheat the oven to 175 ° C (350 ° F).
- Mix the Jamaican spices, salt, and sour cream to make the marinade.
- Pour the mixture into a large plastic sachet with the chicken. Do not take the skin off the chicken!
- Shake vigorously and let marinate for 15 minutes.
- Remove the chicken from the sachet. Bounce the sachet with the marinade.
- Put the chicken in another new and clean bag.
- Undo the pork rinds in fine crumbs in a blender or food processor. Add the coconut flakes and process for a few seconds more.
- Put the crumbs in the new bag with the chicken and stir vigorously.
- Place the chicken in a greased baking sheet, and preferably put it in the oven on a tray that has the

shape of a grill. A "broiler" tray is also a good option.

- Pour olive oil over the chicken. Bake for 40-45 minutes or until the chicken is fully cooked.
- Turn the chicken over after half the time. If the coverage already has a golden color, lower the temperature. The coconut flakes burn easily.
- Meanwhile, prepare the cole slaw. Cut the cabbage into strips with a sharp knife, a mandolin slicer or in a food processor.
- Put the cabbage in a bowl and add salt, pepper and mayonnaise. Mix well and let stand for 10 minutes.

DAY FOUR

BREAKFAST
(Bulletproof Coffee)

A few sips of this emulsion of hot keto coffee , and you'll be ready to face the world. Bulletproof and delicious. Stuff it!

INGREDIENTS
- 240 ml hot coffee, freshly made
- 1 tbsp (15 g) coconut oil
- 1 tbsp unsalted butter

INSTRUCTIONS
- Combine all the ingredients in a blender. Blend until smooth and frothy.
- Serve immediately.
-

ADVICE!
It also works with hot tea, so try it ... a very low carb aftertaste!

LUNCH
(Deep Dish Of Chicken Fajitas)

Is this dish a hot and substantial keto meal or is it a fresh salad? The answer: both! It is also keto , totally tasty and has all the familiar flavors of Tex-Mex cuisine.

INGREDIENTS
- 1 yellow onion
- 1 green paprika
- 75 g butter
- 650 g boneless chicken thighs
- 2 tbsp spice mix tex mex
- 275 g romaine lettuce
- 150 g Mexican cheese
- 2 avocados
- 150 g cherry tomatoes
- 4 tbsp (4 g) fresh coriander
- Salt and ground black pepper
- 225 ml sour cream (optional)

INSTRUCTIONS
- Prepare the garnishes. Chop the lettuce, tomatoes and avocados. Reserve.
- Cut the onion and paprika into thin slices.
- With another knife and different cutting board, cut the chicken into thin pieces.
- Fry the chicken in butter in a large skillet over medium-high heat. Salt and pepper to taste. When

the chicken is almost done, add the onion, paprika and Tex-Mex spice mix.

- Lower the heat and continue frying the mixture while stirring it for a couple of minutes, until the chicken is cooked completely and the vegetables are a little soft.
- Put the lettuce in a bowl and add the chicken, onion and paprika. Put the grated cheese, the avocado and the chopped tomato on top and top with the fresh cilantro and maybe a spoonful of sour cream.

DINNER
(Ketogenic Pizza)

Let us introduce you: pizza, keto , keto, pizza ... This simple recipe is a great way to enjoy a pizza without carbohydrates. It has everything important: pepperoni, cheese and tomato sauce. Delicious!

INGREDIENTS

Base

- 4 eggs
- 175 g grated cheese, preferably mozzarella or provolone
- Coverage
- 3 tbsp tomato concentrate
- 1 tsp Dried oregano

- 120 g grated cheese
- 50 g pepperoni
- black olives

At your service

- 150 g green leafy vegetables
- 4 tbsp olive oil
- sea salt and ground black pepper
-

INSTRUCTIONS

- Preheat the oven to 200 ° C (400 ° F).
- Beat the eggs and add the cheese to the base. Spread this dough on a baking sheet covered with baking paper. You can form two round circles and simply make a large pizza in the shape of a rectangle. Bake 15 minutes until the base turns golden. Remove from the oven and let it cool for a couple of minutes.
- Raise the oven temperature to 225 ° C (450 ° F).
- Spread the tomato concentrate on the base and sprinkle oregano on top. Add cheese on top and top with pepperoni and olives.
- Bake for another 5-10 minutes or until the pizza is browned.
- Serve with a salad.
- advice
- Instead of tomato concentrate, you can also use dried tomato pesto or a jar of pizza sauce or pasta, but make sure it does not contain sugar.

- There are infinite ketogenic ingredients that you can use on pizza: bacon, salami, mushrooms, blue cheese, shredded chicken, sauteed onions, feta cheese ... you know what you like!

DAY FIVE

BREAKFAST
(Omelet Of Keto Cheese)

Do you have cheese, eggs and butter? Then you can improvise something delicious in a short time. Whether it's breakfast, lunch or dinner, this keto dish with a lot of cheese never disappoints. Delight your palate and keep your belly full for hours!

INGREDIENTS

- 75 g butter
- 6 eggs
- 200 g shredded cheddar cheese
- Salt and black pepper ground to taste

INSTRUCTIONS

- Beat the eggs until soft and lightly frothy. Add half of the grated cheddar cheese and mix. Salt and pepper to taste.
- Melt the butter in a hot pan. Pour the egg mixture and let stand for a few minutes.
- Lower the heat and continue cooking until the egg mixture is almost done. Add the remaining grated cheese. Fold and serve immediately.
- Advice!

- Flavor your creation with herbs, chopped vegetables or even Mexican sauce. And do not hesitate to cook the tortilla in olive oil or coconut oil to have a different flavor profile.
- Are you interested in more vegetarian dishes with eggs? Check out our Mexican scrambled eggs , keto frittata with mushrooms and cheese   or classic scrambled eggs .

LUNCH
(Fried Keto Cheese With Mushrooms)

Four ingredients, some seasoning and 15 minutes is all you need to make a delicious vegetarian keto meal that fills a lot.

INGREDIENTS
- 300 g mushrooms
- 300 g halloumi cheese
- 75 g butter
- 10 green olives
- Salt and ground black pepper
- 125 ml (125 g) mayonnaise (optional)

INSTRUCTIONS
- Rinse and cut the mushrooms and chop them or cut them into slices.

- Heat a good amount of butter in a pan where they fit and the halloumi cheese and mushrooms.
- Fry the mushrooms on medium heat for 3-5 minutes until golden brown. Season them.
- If necessary, add more butter and fry the halloumi cheese for a couple of minutes on each side. Stir the mushrooms from time to time. Lower the fire towards the end. Serve with olives.

TIPS!

If halloumi cheese is not available where you live, or if it is very expensive, any hard criollo cheese that does not melt when frying works wonders in this recipe.

This keto dish can be prepared with other low-carb vegetables such as zucchini, asparagus, broccoli and spinach. You can use your favorite seasonings to give more flavor to the dish: ají or paprika powder, some mixture of dried herbs, or perhaps onion, garlic or ground basil.

DINNER
(Keto Burgers With Creamy Tomato Sauce And Fried Cabbage)

A good hamburger does not need any muffins! Enjoy this delicious single burger with a creamy tomato sauce and a garnish of fried cabbage. Keto satisfaction guaranteed!

INGREDIENTS
burgers
- 700 g ground beef
- 1 egg
- 90 g feta cheese
- 1 tsp Salt
- ¼ tsp. ground black pepper
- 50 g fresh parsley, finely chopped
- 1 tbsp olive oil
- 30 g butter

sauce
- 300 ml whipping cream
- 50 g fresh parsley, thickly chopped
- 2 tbsp tomato concentrate
- Salt and ground black pepper

Fried green cabbage
- 700 g grated green cabbage
- 120 g butter
- Salt and ground black pepper

INSTRUCTIONS

- Mix all the ingredients for the burgers and assemble eight of them, longer than wide.
- Fry them over medium heat in butter and olive oil for at least 10 minutes or until the burgers have an appetizing color.
- Pour the tomato concentrate and the cream to beat in the pan when the burgers are almost ready. Mix and let the cream reduce boiling.
- Sprinkle chopped parsley over before serving.
- Green cabbage fried in butter
- Cut the cabbage into strips or use a food processor.
- Melt the butter in a pan.
- Sauté the cabbage in strips over medium heat for at least 15 minutes or until the cabbage acquires the desired color and texture.
- Mix frequently and lower the fire a little towards the end. Salt and pepper to taste.

ADVICE!
Give it a change once in a while! These burgers go well with any vegetable sautéed ... What do you love? Onion, mushrooms, spinach, Brussels sprouts, asparagus, green beans ... As you want!

DAY SIX

BREAKFAST
(Omelet Caprese)

Soft mozzarella, ripe tomatoes and fresh basil? Yes please! And in an omelet - better yet! This easy ketogenic dish works great for breakfast, lunch or dinner and will undoubtedly be one of our favorites.

INGREDIENTS
- 2 tbsp olive oil
- 6 eggs
- 100 g cherry tomatoes cut in halves or tomatoes cut into slices
- 1 tbsp fresh basil or dried basil
- 150 g (325 ml) fresh mozzarella cheese
- salt and pepper

INSTRUCTIONS
- Break the eggs in a bowl to mix and add salt and black pepper to taste. Beat well with a fork until everything is completely mixed. Add basil and stir.
- Cut the tomatoes into halves or slices. Chop or slice the cheese.
- Heat the oil in a large skillet. Fry the tomatoes for a few minutes.
- Pour the egg mixture over the tomatoes. Wait until it becomes a little firm and add the cheese.

- Lower the heat and let the omelet harden. Serve immediately, and enjoy!

LUNCH
(Scrambled Keto Of Cabbage In The Asian Style)

This scrambled keto is so addictive that it is sometimes called "crackslaw" in English. Well, it's so tasty and easy to prepare that it's not surprising! And it's a healthy addiction ..

INGREDIENTS
- 750 g green cabbage
- 150 g butter
- 600 g ground beef
- 1 tsp Salt
- 1 tsp ground onion
- ¼ tsp. ground black pepper
- 1 tbsp White wine vinegar
- 2 cloves of garlic
- 3 chives, chopped
- 1 tsp chili flakes
- 1 tbsp fresh ginger, finely chopped or grated
- 1 tbsp Sesame oil

Wasabi Mayonnaise
- 225 ml (200 g) mayonnaise

- ½ - 1 tbsp wasabi

INSTRUCTIONS
- Cut the cabbage into strips with a sharp knife or food processor.
- Fry the cabbage in 60-90 g (2-3 ounces) of butter in a large skillet or a wok over medium heat but without letting it brown. It takes a long time for the cabbage to soften.
- Add spices and vinegar. Mix and fry for a few more minutes. Put the cabbage in a bowl.
- Melt the rest of the butter in the same pan. Add the chili flakes and the ginger and sauté for a few minutes.
- Add the ground meat and brown it until the meat is fully cooked and most of the juices have evaporated. Lower the fire a little.
- Add the chives and cabbage to the meat and mix until everything has warmed. Season to taste and pour the sesame oil over before serving.
- Assemble the wasabi mayonnaise by mixing a little wasabi in the mayonnaise and adding more until the proper flavor is achieved. Serve the scrambled hot with a good portion of wasabi mayonnaise on top.
- Advice!
- Do you want variety? Replace beef with ground chicken, pork or lamb.

DINNER
(Keto Stew Of Cordon Bleu)

All the flavor, none of the problems. Savor the classic cordon bleu chicken in an instant with this creamy stew, simple to prepare and ketogenic .French style without cooking classes.

Ingredients
- 1 grilled chicken
- 200 g chopped smoked ham
- 200 g (200 ml) cream cheese
- 1 tbsp Dijon mustard
- 1 tbsp white vinegar 5%
- 300 g grated cheddar cheese
- Salt and ground black pepper

At your service
- 150 g lettuce
- 4 tbsp olive oil

INSTRUCTIONS
- Preheat the oven to 200 ° C (400 ° F).
- Cut the cooked chicken and smoked ham into bite-sized pieces.
- Mix the cream cheese, mustard, vinegar and 2/3 of the grated cheese in a greased baking dish. Add the chicken and ham.
- Season to taste and cover with the remaining cheese.
- Bake for 15-20 minutes or until the stew is browned on top.

- Serve with lettuce and olive oil.

ADVICE!
Do not forget to look at the ham label if you buy it from the supermarket: it does not contain sugar!

DAY SEVEN

BREAKFAST
(Keto Stuffed Avocados With Smoked Salmon)

Avocado + smoked salmon = no need to cook. This creamy dish can be eaten at any time of the day and is both exquisitely luxurious and conveniently quick to prepare. You can also serve it as an appetizer at your next dinner with guests. It is simple, tasty, and ketogenic .

INGREDIENTS
- 2 avocados
- 175 g smoked salmon
- 175 ml fresh cream or mayonnaise
- salt and pepper
- 2 tbsp lemon juice (optional)

INSTRUCTIONS
- Cut the avocados in half and remove the bone.
- Put a spoonful of fresh cream in the hollow of the avocado and add smoked salmon on top.
- Season to taste with salt and sprinkle with lemon juice to give more flavor (and avoid the avocado acquires a brown color).
- advice
- This ketogenic dish can be served with any other type of fatty fish, boiled, fried or smoked. It tastes even better with a little fresh dill!

LUNCH
(Keto Dish: The Tex-Mex Burger)

It's about authentic food on a plate.A hamburger, cheese, arugula and avocado. Because a ketogenic food does not have to be complicated.

INGREDIENTS
- 300 g ground beef
- 2 tbsp cold water
- 1 tbsp spice mix tex mex
- 2 tbsp jalapeños in vinegar
- 125 ml fresh cream or mayonnaise
- 120 g Mexican cheese, sliced
- 2 avocados
- 50 g rocket
- 2 tbsp olive oil
- Salt and ground black pepper

INSTRUCTIONS
- Mix ground beef, Tex-Mex spice mix and water. Assemble one hamburger per serving.
- Apply olive oil with a brush all over the surface of each burger. Fry or grill them 3-4 minutes on each side until they become light pink or fully cooked, whichever you prefer.
- Salt and pepper to taste. Place the hamburger on a plate with avocado, lettuce, jalapeños and fresh cream

or mayonnaise. Spray olive oil on the vegetables.
- advice
- Give it a spicier touch with our keto green sauce , it's delicious with the avocado!

DINNER
(Keto Chicken With Herb Butter)

This keto meal is so delicious and so quick to prepare that you will sing praises to anyone who wants to listen! Melt a good portion of butter on this delicious chicken, fried also in butter. It's a butter party and, well, you're going to enjoy it!

INGREDIENTS
Fried chicken
- 4 chicken breasts
- 30 g butter or olive oil
- Salt and ground black pepper
Herbal butter
- 150 g butter, at room temperature
- 1 clove of garlic
- ½ tsp. garlic powder
- 60 ml fresh chopped parsley
- 1 tsp lemon juice
- ½ tsp. Salt

Green leafy vegetables
225 g green leafy vegetables, for example spinach sprouts

INSTRUCTIONS
- Remove the butter from the refrigerator so that it acquires the room temperature.
- Start with the herb butter. Mix all the ingredients in a small bowl until they are completely incorporated. Let rest until serving time.
- Season the chicken. Fry in butter or oil over medium heat until fillets are fully cooked and have a temperature of 75 ° C (165 ° F) when measured with a meat thermometer. Lower the fire towards the end to prevent the fillets from drying out.
- Serve the chicken over green leafy vegetables and top with a good portion of herbed butter.

ADVICE!
It's easy to always have this delicious herb butter on hand! You can prepare it in advance and store it in the refrigerator for up to 3 days.And it is super versatile. Combine perfectly with other meat dishes: try it with beef or turkey or pork chops.

DAY EIGHT

BREAKFAST
(The Classic Bacon With Eggs)

It is one of the best ketogenic breakfasts that exist! Make this classic something even more delicious with this wonderful recipe.Enjoy the amount of eggs you need to satisfy yourself, depending on your level of hunger. Just thinking about this keto dish makes our mouth water!

INGREDIENTS
- 8 eggs
- 150 g bacon, sliced
- cherry tomato (optional)
- fresh parsley (optional)

INSTRUCTIONS
- Fry the bacon until crispy. Set aside on a plate.
- Fry the eggs in the bacon fat the way you like. Cut the cherry tomatoes in half and fry them at the same time.
- Salt and pepper to taste.

ADVICE!
If you can, try using organic bacon ... it's healthier and contains fewer additives.

LUNCH
(Caesar Keto Salad)

An authentic classic salad made keto . In our version, you do not need to skimp on salsa or Parmesan cheese!

INGREDIENTS
- 300 g chicken breasts
- 1 tbsp olive oil
- Salt and ground black pepper
- 150 g bacon
- ½ romaine lettuce
- 50 g freshly grated parmesan cheese

Dressing
- 125 ml (125 g) mayonnaise
- 1 tbsp Dijon mustard
- ½ lemon, juice and grated rind
- 2 tbsp grated Parmesan cheese
- 2 tbsp Anchovy fillets, finely chopped
- Salt and ground black pepper

INSTRUCTIONS
- Mix the ingredients for the dressing with a whisk or an electric mixer. Put aside in the refrigerator.
- Preheat the oven to 200 ° C (400 ° F). Place the chicken breasts in a greased baking dish.

- Season the chicken and sprinkle with olive oil or melted butter. Bake for 20 minutes or until cooked through. You can also cook the chicken in the burners, if you prefer.
- Fry the bacon until crispy. Cut the lettuce into strips and put it on two plates. Put the chicken on top and then add the crumbled bacon.
- Top with a good dose of dressing and Parmesan cheese.

ADVICE!

This recipe works wonders when there is more than enough roast chicken from another meal, or with grilled chicken that is bought from the supermarket.

DINNER
(Creamy Ketogenic Fish Casserole)

A plate of white fish bathed in a creamy sauce becomes even more flavorful with the salty touch of capers and the freshness of broccoli and green leafy vegetables. Impossible to find an easier dinner than this all-in-one wonder!

INGREDIENTS
- 2 tbsp olive oil
- 450 g broccoli
- 6 chives
- 2 tbsp small capers
- 30 g butter, to grease the asadera

- 700 g white fish, in the size of individual portions
- 300 ml whipping cream
- 1 tbsp Dijon mustard
- 1 tsp Salt
- ¼ tsp. ground black pepper
- 1 tbsp dry parsley
- 90 g butter

For serving
- 150 g green leafy vegetables

INSTRUCTIONS
- Preheat the oven to 200 ° C (400 ° F).
- Separate the broccoli into small twigs, including the stem. Peel the stem with a sharp knife or a potato peeler if it is very rough.
- Fry the broccoli in oil over medium heat for 5 minutes until it becomes soft and golden. Pepper.
- Add the chives, finely chopped, and the capers.Fry another 1-2 minutes more and put the vegetables in a greased baking sheet.
- Place the fish between the vegetables.
- Mix the parsley, the whipping cream and the mustard. Pour the mixture over the fish with vegetables. Top with slices of butter.
- Bake for 20 minutes or until the fish is fully cooked and easily peeled with a fork. Serve it like that or with a tasty green salad.

ADVICE!

You can give it some variety using salmon or tuna (fresh or frozen) instead of white fish. The trout works great too if you do not have access to salmon. Or if you hate broccoli, you can substitute Brussels sprouts, asparagus, zucchini or mushrooms. If you use your imagination, you will never get bored of this all-in-one dinner.

DAY NINE

BREAKFAST
(Ketogenic Latte Chai)

Flavor your cup with this warm and aromatic classic. Chai tea, served as a keto- style latte , is perfect for the colder months. A creamy mix that you will love.

INGREDIENTS
- 1 tbsp Chai tea
- 475 ml water
- 75 ml whipping cream

INSTRUCTIONS
- Prepare the tea in hot water according to the package instructions. Make sure you let it taste as much as possible without becoming bitter.
- Heat the cream in the microwave or in a small saucepan and add to the tea before serving.

ADVICE!
Do you want to prepare the rich gingerbread cookies that are in the image? Here is the recipe !

LUNCH
(Keto Dish Of Roast Beef And Cheddar Cheese)

In this recipe it is authentic food on a plate, simple and simple.Roasted meat, cheese, avocado, radishes, chives, and period.Because a ketogenic food does not have to be complicated.

INGREDIENTS
- 200 g cooked beef style cold cuts
- 150 g cheddar cheese
- 1 avocado
- 6 radishes
- 1 scallion
- 125 ml (125 g) mayonnaise
- 1 tbsp Dijon mustard
- 50 g lettuce
- 2 tbsp olive oil
- Salt and ground black pepper

INSTRUCTIONS
- Place the roast beef, cheese, avocado and radishes on a plate.
- Add sliced onion and a good dose of mayonnaise.
- Serve with lettuce and olive oil.

ADVICE
Change a bit of mayonnaise for butter and try the radishes with butter and salt. Simple and delicious!

DINNER
(Keto Chicken Skewers With Fried "Potatoes" And Sauce)

The "potatoes" of this recipe are so crunchy, golden and light that almost remain with all the leading role. But the delicious and quick skewers to prepare - with a good dose of fresh spinach sauce and spreads - are team actors: they do not mind sharing the lead role. Greetings, guys, to your audience: they are a company that really makes a wonderful show. Bis!

INGREDIENTS
Chicken skewers
- 4 - 8 wooden skewers
- 4 chicken breasts
- ½ tsp. Salt
- ¼ tsp. ground black pepper
- 2 tbsp olive oil

Spinach sauce to spread
- 2 tbsp light olive oil
- 50 g frozen spinach, chopped
- 2 tbsp dry parsley
- 1 tbsp dry dill
- 1 tsp ground onion
- ½ tsp. Salt
- ¼ tsp. ground black pepper

- 240 ml (225 g) mayonnaise
- 60 ml sour cream
- 2 tsp lemon juice

"Potatoes" fried with celery roots

- 500 g celery root
- 2 tbsp olive oil
- ½ tsp. Salt
- ¼ tsp. ground black pepper

INSTRUCTIONS

- Prepare the sauce to spread. Thaw spinach and remove excess liquid. Pour into a bowl and mix well with the other ingredients.
- Let it rest in the refrigerator while you prepare the skewers and fried "potatoes".
- Preheat the oven to 200 ° C (400 ° F), using the broil option, if your oven has it.
- Cut the chicken into pieces of 2.5 cm and place it in a bowl or a plastic bag.
- Add spices and oil and mix. Marinate for 5-10 minutes at room temperature. Meanwhile, prepare the fried "potatoes" according to step number 9.
- Puncture the chicken or four skewers, or eight smaller ones. Place them on a baking sheet covered with baking paper.
- Roast for 20-30 minutes or until the chicken is fully cooked. Adjust the time according to the size of the skewers. Keep them warm during the preparation of the "potatoes".

- If you have a convection oven, you can prepare the skewers and the "potatoes" at the same time.
- Peel the celery roots and cut them into strips. Put them in a bowl or plastic bag. Season and add oil. Mix or shake.
- Place them on a baking sheet or in a large roasting pan. Bake for 20 minutes or until they become soft and golden brown.

ADVICE!

Give more variety! Baking skewers is simple and convenient, but do not hesitate to cook them in a pan or put them on the grill. The two techniques provide their own depth of flavor. So choose yourself: which one is your favorite?

DAY TEN

BREAKFAST
(Keto Cheese Rolls)

This is the fastest, simplest and most tasty ketogenic recipe in the world. It is impossible to resist this salty delight!

INGREDIENTS
- 225 g sliced cheddar or provolone cheese or edam cheese
- 60 g butter

INSTRUCTIONS
- Place the slices of cheese on a large cutting board. Cut the butter into thin slices using a slicer for cheese or a knife.
- Put a slice of butter on each slice of cheese and roll. Serve as breakfast or snack.

ADVICE!
These cheese rolls are delicious as they are, but you can also add some extras.For example, combine wonderful paprika powder, flakes of salt, parsley, or other finely chopped herbs.

LUNCH
(Asparagus Wrapped In Cured Ham With Goat Cheese)

Crispy asparagus, creamy goat cheese and salted cured ham come together to create the perfect trio of flavors. This dish is so elegant that you wonder if you should have dressed in full dress. And it's so simple to prepare that it will not cause you any stress. It is an easy recipe that you can prepare any day of the week.

Bjarte , our chief of operations, shared this recipe with us. In your home it is one of the foods that you eat most often.

INGREDIENTS
- 12 green asparagus
- 50 g cured ham, in thin slices
- 150 g goat cheese
- ¼ tsp. ground black pepper
- 2 tbsp olive oil

INSTRUCTIONS
- Preheat the oven to 225 ° C (450 ° F), preferably with the grill on.
- Wash and trim the asparagus.
- Cut the cheese into 12 slices and then divide each slice into two.
- Cut the slices into two pieces along and wrap an asparagus in a piece of cured ham and two pieces of cheese.

- Place them in a baking dish, season with pepper and sprinkle with olive oil.
- Bake for 15 minutes until golden brown.

ADVICE!

Do it the way you like it best! If you follow the recipe, the asparagus will be crunchy but tender. If you prefer that the asparagus be softer, you can scald them for 1-2 minutes.

DINNER
(Ketogenic Frittata With Mushrooms And Cheese)

They are also known as "the open omelet of Italy".The frittatas are easy to prepare and super versatile, you can enjoy them at any time of the day. This version contains fresh mushrooms and cream cheese: bellissimo! They are the perfect complement for eggs in this classic ketogenic dish . Buon appetito !

INGREDIENTS
Frittata
- 450 g mushrooms
- 90 g butter
- 6 chives
- 1 tbsp fresh parsley
- 1 tsp Salt
- ½ tsp. ground black pepper
  10 eggs

- 225 g grated cheese
- 240 ml (225 g) mayonnaise
- 110 g green leafy vegetables

INSTRUCTIONS

- Preheat the oven to 175 ° C (350 ° F). First, prepare the vinaigrette sauce and reserve it.
- Cut the mushrooms in the shape and size you want.
- Sauté the mushrooms over medium heat in most of the butter until golden brown. Lower the fire. Save some butter to grease the broiler pan.
- Chop the chives and mix them with the fried mushrooms. Season to taste and mix with the parsley.
- Mix the eggs, mayonnaise and cheese in a separate bowl. Salt and pepper to taste.
- Add the mushrooms and chives and pour everything into a well-greased roasting pan. Bake for 30-40 minutes or until the frittata turns golden and the eggs are cooked.
- Let it cool for 5 minutes and serve with green leafy vegetables and the vinaigrette sauce.

ADVICE!

Make sure you choose the cheese well! Choose a variety that has a superior melting quality such as cheddar, fontina or gruyere.

DAY ELEVEN

BREAKFAST
(Egg Muffin)

This ketogenic recipe is one of the best to save you time, without a doubt! Muffins are convenient and easy to prepare: perfect for busy adults and children. You can prepare them in advance and give yourself a pat on the back for being so organized!

INGREDIENTS
- 8 eggs
- 1 spring onion, finely chopped
- 150 g dried chorizo with air or salami or cooked bacon
- 75 g grated cheese
- 1 tbsp red pesto or green pesto (optional)
- Salt and ground black pepper

INSTRUCTIONS
- Preheat the oven to 175 ° C (350 ° F).
- Chop the chives and meat finely.
- Beat the eggs together with the condiments and the pesto. Add the cheese and mix.
- Put the dough in muffin molds and add bacon, sausage or salami.

- Bake for 15-20 minutes, depending on the size of the mold.

TIPS!

Kids love these muffins full of cheese.They are perfect to carry in the lunch box.

LUNCH
(Tuna Keto Salad With Hard Boiled Eggs)

Is a keto meal ready in 15 minutes? Yes, please! It is a creamy tuna salad served on crispy lettuce, accompanied with eggs cooked to perfection and a little tomato to give it color. Advantage!

INGREDIENTS
- 110 g (250 ml) branches of celery
- 2 scallions
- 150 g tuna in olive oil
- 175 ml (150 g) mayonnaise
- ½ lemon, juice and grated rind
- 1 tsp Dijon mustard
- 4 eggs
- 225 g romaine lettuce
- 110 g cherry tomatoes
- 2 tbsp olive oil
- Salt and ground black pepper

INSTRUCTIONS

- Chop the celery and chives finely. Add them to a medium bowl with the tuna, lemon, mayonnaise and mustard. Mix to incorporate everything and salt and pepper to taste. Reserve to use later.
- Put the eggs in a pot and add water to cover the eggs. Bring to a boil and simmer for 5-6 minutes (for water-washed eggs) or 8-10 minutes (for hard-boiled eggs).
- When cooked, put them in cold water immediately so they peel more easily. Cut them into wedges or halves.
- Place the tuna mixture and eggs on some romaine lettuce leaves. Add the tomatoes and sprinkle olive oil on top. Salt and pepper to taste.

DINNER
(Keto Curry Casserole With Chicken)

Do you need something to warm yourself? This tasty but simple curry casserole with chicken, cauliflower, and coconut will give it to you! It is a substantial keto meal that is prepared in less than half an hour.

INGREDIENTS

- 650 g boneless chicken thighs

- 1 tbsp curry powder
- 1 tsp garlic powder
- 60 ml (50 g) coconut oil
- 450 g (1 liter) cauliflower
- 1 green paprika
- 400 g coconut milk
- Salt and ground black pepper
- 60 ml (4 g) fresh coriander or fresh parsley

INSTRUCTIONS

- Crumble the chicken and cut the cauliflower and paprika into smaller pieces.
- Heat the coconut oil in a large skillet or wok. Add the curry powder and the ground garlic and fry for a minute to release the flavors.
- Add the shredded chicken and salt and pepper. Fry for about 5 minutes. Stir from time to time to make sure all the pieces are cooked equally.
- Add the cauliflower and the paprika. Cook the vegetables together with the chicken for a few minutes.
- Add the coconut milk and let the casserole simmer for about 5-10 minutes. Season with more salt and pepper.
- Serve with finely chopped coriander on top.

DAY TWELVE

BREAKFAST
(Mexican Scrambled Eggs)

Give your breakfast a spicy touch with this tasty dish keto with eggs.Jalapenos, tomatoes and chives come together to form a perfectly balanced flavor combination. They guarantee to animate your day!

INGREDIENTS
- 6 eggs
- 1 scallion
- 2 jalapenos in vinegar, finely chopped
- 1 tomato, finely chopped
- 75 g grated cheese
- 2 tbsp butter, to fry
- Salt and ground black pepper

INSTRUCTIONS
- Finely chop chives, jalapenos and tomatoes. Fry in butter for 3 minutes over medium heat.
- Beat the eggs and pour them into the pan. Stir them for 2 minutes. Then add the cheese and salt and pepper.
- Advice!

- To add even more life to this meal, serve it with avocado, crispy lettuce and a dressing.

LUNCH
(Keto Ground Beef With Green Beans)

A wonder that is prepared in a single pan: it is authentic food, inexpensive ingredients, simple preparation, delicious food, and easy cleaning. It's fast food Keto prepared right there in your kitchen. Let's go!

INGREDIENTS
- 300 g ground beef
- 250 g fresh green beans
- 100 g butter
- Salt and ground black pepper
- 75 ml (75 g) mayonnaise or fresh cream

INSTRUCTIONS
- Rinse and trim green beans.
- Heat a generous amount of butter in a pan where the ground beef and green beans will enter.
- Brown the ground beef over high heat until it is almost ready. Pepper.
- Lower the heat a little. Add more butter and fry the green beans 5 minutes in the same pan. Stir the ground beef occasionally.
- Season the green beans. Serve with the remaining butter and add mayonnaise or fresh cream if you need

more fat to sate.

ADVICE!
This keto dish can be prepared with other low-carb vegetables too, such as zucchini, asparagus, broccoli or spinach. You can use your favorite seasonings to give more flavor to the dish: chili or paprika powder, or perhaps onion or ground garlic, or some basil.

DINNER
(Sullivan's Keto Pizza)

It is rare that the dough of a keto pizza can be gripped by hand. This pizza dough is even more crunchy than the famous fat head pizza and is perfect to hold with your hands, you do not need a fork or plate!

INGREDIENTS
Base
- 125 ml (100 g) unflavored protein powder (whey)
- ½ tsp. baking powder
- ½ tsp. granulated garlic
- ½ tsp. Salt
- ½ tsp. Italian spices mix
- 75 g grated parmesan cheese
- 75 g (150 ml) mozzarella cheese
- 50 g (50 ml) cream cheese
- 4 tbsp olive oil
- 1 egg

Ingredients on the basis

- 60 ml tomato sauce without sugar
- 225 g shredded cheddar cheese
- ½ red pepper
- 225 g Italian sausages
- 1 tbsp chopped fresh basil

INSTRUCTIONS

- Preheat the oven to 190 ° C (375 ° F).
- Combine all the ingredients in a large bowl to mix. The mass will be thicker than a malleable mass.
- Line a baking sheet or a pizza stone with baking paper. Use a spoon or a wooden pallet to smooth the dough until it is round and about 22 cm. You can also divide the dough into quarters and create four of 13 cm (5 inches) (if you make 4 servings).
- Bake the dough for 9 to 12 minutes or until golden brown.
- Remove from the oven, cover with tomato sauce and your favorite pizza ingredients or reserve the masses to use later.
- After pouring the ingredients, put it in the oven to bake until the ingredients are golden and the cheese melted.

TIPS

These doughs freeze very well and can be removed from the freezer, place the ingredients and then baked until hot for a quick pizza meal. Kristie's favorite low-carb ingredients are:

sausages, pepperoni, peppers, onions, bacon, black olives and mozzarella cheese.

DAY THIRTEEN

BREAKFAST
(Halloumi Cheese Wrapped In Bacon)

Salty cheese wrapped in salty bacon? We signed up! Serve these delicious keto bites on lettuce and green leafy vegetables, and it will be the best salad you've ever tasted!

INGREDIENTS
- 225 g halloumi cheese
- 150 g bacon, sliced

INSTRUCTIONS
- Preheat the oven to 225 ° C (450 ° F).
- Cut the cheese into 8-10 pieces.
- Wrap each piece of cheese in a slice of bacon.
- Place them on a baking sheet and put them in the oven for 10-15 minutes, or until golden brown. Turn them around when half the time has passed.

ADVICE!
Are you reluctant to light the oven tonight?You can fry the cheese in a pan over medium heat with a little oil or butter. If you want to vary it, you can use pancetta instead of bacon.

Do you crave an extra explosion of flavors and textures? A sauce to spread is just what you need! Here you can see our seasoning recipes !

LUNCH
(Keto Zucchini Rolls With Chorizo)

Use the right amount of spices with this tasty food. Zucchini and mushrooms mark the way, but the touch of chorizo reaches the palate. One of our favorite keto dishes with a cheese flavor that can be eaten alone or enjoyed as a garnish.

INGREDIENTS
- 700 g zucchini
- ½ tsp. Salt
- 90 g butter
- 175 g mushrooms, finely chopped
- 175 g (175 ml) cream cheese
- 175 g grated cheese
- ½ green pepper, finely chopped
- 75 g dried chorizo with air
- 1 egg
- 1 tsp ground onion
- 2 tbsp fresh parsley, chopped
- ½ tsp. Salt
- ¼ tsp. ground black pepper
- 240 ml (225 g) mayonnaise or butter with herbs, to serve

- 50 g green leafy vegetables, to serve

INSTRUCTIONS

- Preheat the oven to 175 ° C (350 ° F). Cut the zucchini longitudinally into slices of 1 centimeter and quarter and place in a baking sheet lined with baking paper.
- Pour salt and let stand for ten minutes. Dry the liquid with a paper towel or a clean kitchen towel.
- Bake for 20 minutes or until the zucchini is soft. Remove from the oven and let cool on a grill.
- Chop and fry the mushrooms in butter until well browned. Let cool.
- Place all the other ingredients, except for a third of the grated cheese, in a bowl. Add the mushrooms and mix well.
- Place a generous amount of cheese dough on top of each zucchini slice.
- Roll each slice and place the rolls with the closure facing down in a greased baking dish. Sprinkle the rest of the cheese on top.
- Increase the temperature to 200 ° C (400 ° F). Bake for 20-30 minutes or until golden brown on top.
- Serve with mayonnaise and green leafy vegetables.

ADVICE!

Do not hesitate to try this recipe with different cheeses to have other flavors.You can also make this dish with eggplant instead of zucchini.

DINNER
(Pork Chops With Green Beans And Garlic Butter)

Juicy pork chops, crispy green beans, and garlic butter ... This is a wonder, and it is prepared in a pan. It is keto elegance at its best.

INGREDIENTS
- 4 pork chops
- 50 g butter, for frying
- 450 g fresh green beans
- Salt and ground black pepper

Garlic butter
- 150 g butter, at room temperature
- 1 tbsp dry parsley
- ½ cda. garlic powder
- 1 tbsp lemon juice
- Salt and ground black pepper

INSTRUCTIONS
- Remove the butter from the refrigerator and allow it to rise to a room temperature.
- Mix butter, garlic, parsley and lemon juice. Salt and pepper to taste. Reserve.
- Make a few small cuts in the fat around the chops so they stay flat when cold. Salt and pepper to taste.

- Heat a skillet over medium-high heat. Add the butter, then the chops.
- Fry the chops for about 5 minutes on each side until they are golden brown and fully cooked.
- Remove the chops from the pan and keep them warm.
- Use the same pan and add the green beans. Salt and pepper to taste. Cook over medium-high heat for a couple of minutes until the beans get a bright color and are a little soft, but still crispy.
- Serve chops and green beans with a good portion of melted butter on top.

ADVICE!

You can use green beans frozen or canned. They are not as crispy as fresh ones, but still have a good flavor and it is easy to store them in the refrigerator or pantry.

DAY FOURTEEN

BREAKFAST
(Scrambled Eggs)

Butter + eggs = the perfect ketogenic breakfast. This is how the day begins, with a particularly delicious and buttery version of this classic breakfast. And it's ready in just a few minutes!

INGREDIENTS
- 2 eggs
- 30 g butter
- Salt and ground black pepper

INSTRUCTIONS
- Beat the eggs together with some salt and pepper using a fork.
- Melt the butter in a nonstick skillet over medium heat. Look closely: butter does not turn golden!
- Pour the eggs into the pan and mix for 1-2 minutes until they are creamy and cooked a little less than you like. Remember that the eggs will continue to cook even once you put them on your plate.

TIPS!
These creamy eggs pair well with many popular low carb dishes. Of course, there is the option of eating them with

classic accompaniments such as bacon or sausage, but there are other great options such as salmon, avocado, cold cuts and cheese (cheddar, fresh mozzarella or feta).

LUNCH
(Keto Burgers Wrapped In Bacon)

Why not? The burgers combine wonderfully with the bacon. You can put some together tonight and become the brilliant cook you always wanted to be. This dish is loaded with all the favorite ingredients and everyone will love it.

INGREDIENTS
- 200 g bacon
- 600 g ground beef
- 2 tbsp cold water
- 2 tsp chili paste
- 1 tsp garlic powder or ground onion (optional)
- ½ tsp. Salt
- ½ tsp. ground black pepper
- 1 tbsp olive oil

At your service
- 75 g Pickled cucumbers with dill
- 75 g sliced cheddar cheese
- 75 g lettuce
- 2 tomatoes cut into slices

- 1 red onion cut into slices
- 150 ml (150 g) mayonnaise

INSTRUCTIONS

- Reserve a slice of bacon for each burger and chop the remaining slices.
- Mix ground beef, water, chili paste, chopped bacon and spices. Arrange the hamburgers with wet hands.
- Wrap each hamburger in a slice of bacon. Apply the olive oil to the meat with a brush and grill for 5-10 minutes on each side.
- Serve with cheddar cheese, pickles, lettuce, tomato, onion and a good dose of mayonnaise.

ADVICE

Have fun and vary the type of ground beef you use. Both the lamb and the turkey go well with the bacon.Using a mixture of ground beef and pork can be wonderful, if you find it. And do not hesitate to add finely chopped herbs: rosemary and oregano are an excellent complement to the flavors of meat.

Do not forget the condiments! Our homemade ketchup is totally natural and sugar free, and is one of our most popular recipes: why not try it today?

DINNER
(Buffalo-Style Chicken With Paprika Mayonnaise And Fried Cabbage In Butter)

These juicy chicken prey have just the right amount of spiciness and are served with a mild but tasty paprika mayonnaise and fried cabbage in butter. It is a ketogenic food that you will want to prepare over and over again.

INGREDIENTS
- 800 g chicken thighs
- 2 tbsp hot sauce
- 3 tbsp olive oil
- 1 tbsp garlic powder
- 1 tsp Salt

Fried cabbage in butter
- 650 g green cabbage
- 50 g butter
- Salt and ground black pepper

Paprika Mayonnaise
- 175 ml (150 g) mayonnaise
- 1 tbsp Spanish paprika
- ½ tsp. hot sauce
- Salt and ground black pepper

INSTRUCTIONS
- Preheat the oven to 200 ° C (400 ° F).
- Mix olive oil, garlic powder, hot sauce and salt in a large bowl.
- Add the thighs and stir in the mixture to cover them. Alternatively, apply the mixture to the thighs with a brush.

- Put the chicken in a greased baking sheet with the skin facing upwards.
- Bake for 40 minutes or until the chicken is fully cooked. If you use a thermometer, the chicken will be ready when it shows a value of 82 ° C (180 ° F).
- In a small bowl, mix the mayonnaise, the paprika powder and the spicy sauce or tabasco. Reserve.
- Cut the cabbage into thin strips with a knife or food processor.
- Fry the cabbage in a pan over medium heat until it is soft, and golden on the edges. Salt and pepper to taste.
- Serve the chicken and cabbage with a good dose of flavored mayonnaise and maybe an extra pinch of hot sauce.

NOTE

Do not hesitate to adjust this menu meal plan according to your tastes.

Intermittent Fasting: TheStrategy To Lose Weight And What Science Says About It

According to the latest and most important meta-analyses, fasting is a very useful tool in nutrition. Under this premise appear dietary strategies such as intermittent fasting. How useful are they and what are they based on?Scientific evidence supports the usefulness of fasting in many cases.

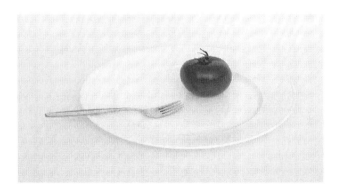

Fasting has the scientific endorsement

The myth that it is healthier to eat five times a day is widespread. This is based on a misconception that not going hungry is healthier since it does not force the body to "save reserves." However, nothing supports this concept. Quite the contrary. A recent meta-analysis, which analyzes a large part of the scientific literature published on the subject to date, indicated that the number of intakes has no benefit.However, reduce meals and leave a space of several hours between them (in other words, fast) yes. This review analyzes several fasting systems and the evidence that support them. The conclusions reached are that the temporary caloric restriction helps to reduce the risk factors of several diseases, among which include the metabolic syndrome, cardiovascular diseases, cancer, and even neurodegenerative diseases.

Other studies also suggest that reducing the time of intake, and spacing between meals, helps reduce body fat, increase the amount of lean mass (muscle), reduce metabolic age and even help with neuroplasticity. All these results are consistent with the conclusions of the meta-analysis that we mentioned, although this focuses more on vascular and metabolic diseases in adults. Despite the growing amount of information about fasting, almost all studies agree that more information is needed.

How does intermittent fasting work?

From the evidence on fasting, some experts in nutrition and sports preparation design strategies to take advantage of their benefits. Intermittent fasting, or Intermittent Fasting (IF), consists of alternating periods without eating with periods of intake at specific times. The best known are fasting 16/8, 24 and 48, but they are not the only ones.With these figures, reference is made to the time between intakes. Thus, fasting 16/8 consists of fasting periods of 16 hours, followed by periods in which we can eat normally for eight hours. If, for example, we carry out the first meal at 2:00

p.m., we can eat until 10:00 p.m., for 8 hours.From then on, we would keep fasting until 2:00 pm the next day, 16 hours later. You can eat normally and as many times as you want during these eight hours of intake, although this increases the risk of eating more calories than we would eat in a single meal.

It is necessary to clarify that the period of intake is not synonymous with having carte blanche to eat anything and in any way. If we want to lose weight, we must maintain a hypocaloric diet. This must be well structured nutritionally speaking, to avoid problems of malnutrition. The idea is to base our diet on healthy foods and not on ultra-processed products, which contain a poor nutritional value. For daily fasts, the strategy consists of eating for 24 hours, fasting other 24, etc. In short, according to the results of the meta-analysis that we mentioned, the important thing is to consume almost the entire diet in a short period of the day, between 4 and 12 hours. It is not necessary to reduce the number of calories we eat, although it is essential to eat healthy, of course.This means fasting for 12 or 20 hours in a row , which is the period analyzed that benefits the most, according to the studies. For example, we could eat for 12 hours and fast for another 12 overtaking dinner and delaying breakfast . The researchers conclude that stopping eating between these 12 and 20 hours can help improve body weight, fat and muscle composition as well as reduce various processes associated with the disease.

Myths About Diets And Weight Loss

Myth: Fad diets are a good way for me to lose weight and not increase it again.

Truth: Fad diets are not the best way to lose weight permanently. This type of diet generally promises that you will lose weight quickly. They make you strictly reduce what you eat or avoid certain types of foods. It is possible that at first you lose weight, but it is difficult to continue this type of diet.Most people soon tire of following them and regain the weight they had lost.Some fad diets are not healthy and do not provide all the nutrients the body needs. Also, if you lose more than 3 pounds (almost 1½ kilos) a week for several weeks, you may increase the chance that you will develop gallstones (masses of solid material in the gallbladder that can be painful). If you follow a diet of less than 800 calories a day for a long time, you may have serious heart problems.

 Tip: Research suggests that the safest way to lose weight and not increase weight again is by following a healthy diet with fewer calories than what you used to eat and exercising every day. The goal is to lose from ½ pound to 2 pound (from ¼ kilo to 1 kilo) per week (after the first weeks of weight loss).Choose healthy foods Eat small portions.Incorporate exercise into your daily routine. Together, these eating and exercise habits can be a healthy way to lose weight and not increase it again. These habits also decrease your chance of developing heart disease, high blood pressure and type 2 diabetes.

Myth: Grain products such as bread, pasta and rice make me fat. I must avoid them when I try to lose weight.

Truth: A grain product is any food that is made with wheat, rice, oats, barley or other cereal. The grains are divided into two subgroups: whole grains and refined grains. Whole grains contain all the germ of the seed-the bran, the germ and the endosperm.Some examples are brown rice and whole wheat bread, cereals and pasta.The refined grains have been ground, a process through which the bran and germ are removed.This is done to give the grains a finer texture and increases the shelf life of the perishable products, however, it removes dietary fiber, iron and many of the B vitamins.

It is possible that people who eat whole grains as part of a healthy diet reduce their chances of developing some chronic diseases. Government dietary guidelines suggest that half of the grains you consume are whole grains.For example, select bread that has 100 percent whole wheat flour instead of white bread, and brown rice instead of white rice.Additional links to these guidelines and the MyPlate website are provided in the Additional Information section at the end of this sheet., which provides information, practical suggestions and tools to eat healthy.

Tip: To lose weight, you have to eat fewer calories and increase the amount of exercise or physical activity you do each day. Establish and follow a healthy eating plan that replaces less healthy options with a mix of fruits, vegetables, whole grains, protein foods and low-fat dairy products:

- Eat a variety of fruits, vegetables, whole grains, and milk and its fat-free or low-fat dairy products.
- Limit added sugars, cholesterol, salt (sodium) and saturated fats, also known as "solid fats," which are the fats that come from fatty meats and high-fat dairy products like butter .
- Eat protein that is low in fat such as beans, eggs, fish, lean meats, nuts, and chicken or turkey.

Eat vegetables and fruits of all colors!

When you fill half of your plate with fruits and vegetables, choose foods with a diversity of intense colors. So you will get a variety of vitamins, minerals and fiber.

- Red red peppers, cherries, cranberries, red onions, beets (beetroot or beet), strawberries, tomatoes, watermelon
- Green avocados, broccoli, cabbage, cucumbers, dark lettuce, grapes, green melon, kale, kiwis, spinach, Italian green zucchini ("zuchinni")
- Orange and yellow apricots, bananas or bananas, melons, papaya, carrots, mangoes, oranges, peaches or peaches, pumpkins, sweet potatoes (sweet potato or sweet potato)

- Blue and purple blackberries, blueberries (blue berries), grapes, plums, purple cabbage, purple carrots, purple potatoes

Myth: Some people can eat everything they want and still lose weight.

Truth: To lose weight, you need to burn more calories than you eat and drink. There are people who look like they can eat any type of food they want and still lose weight.However, like other people, in order to lose weight, they have to use more energy than they ingest through food.There are some factors that can affect your weight.These include age, medications, the habits of daily life and the genes you inherited from your parents. If you want to lose weight, talk with your doctor about the factors that can affect your weight. Together you can create a plan for you to achieve your weight and health goals.

Tip: Just because you are trying to lose weight, it does not mean that you can not eat your favorite foods. The important thing is that you have a healthy eating plan and if one day you eat something that fattens a lot, that is, that has many calories, try to eat less the rest of the day or the next day. For this it is good to look at the total number of calories you eat and reduce the size of your portions. Find how to limit calories in your favorite foods. For example, you can bake some foods instead of frying them or you can use low-fat milk instead of cream. Do not forget to fill half of your plate with fruits and vegetables.

Myth: I should not eat fast foods when I'm dieting because they're an unhealthy selection.

Truth: It is true that many fast foods are not very healthy and can make you gain weight. However, if you are in a place where fast foods are served, select the menu options carefully. Both at home and on the street, choose small portions of healthy foods that are high in nutrients and low in calories.

Tip: To choose healthy and low-calorie foods, review the nutritional data. Today you can often find them on menus or on restaurant websites. However, do not forget that nutritional information does not always include sauces or extras. Try these tips:

- Avoid combos or specials, which despite giving you more for your money, tend to have more calories than you need in a single meal.
- Choose fresh fruit or non-fat yogurt for dessert.
- Limit the use of extra ingredients that are high in fat and calories, such as bacon, cheese, regular mayonnaise, salad dressings, and tartar sauce.
- Choose products that are steamed, grilled or baked instead of fried. For example, try chicken breast to griddle instead of fried chicken.
- Drink water or milk without fat instead of soda.
- As a companion, serve a salad or a small portion of rice with beans instead of cassava or potato chips.

Myth: If I miss a meal, I can lose weight.

Truth: If you skip a meal, you may end up feeling more hungry. This can make you eat more than usual at the next meal. Studies show a relationship between not eating breakfast and obesity. People who do not eat breakfast often weigh more than people who eat a healthy breakfast.

  Tip: Choose foods and snacks that include a variety of healthy foods. Try the following examples:

- Quick breakfast: Eat oatmeal with low-fat milk and top it with fresh fruit or eat whole-wheat toast with fruit jam.
- Healthy lunches: prepare your lunch every night, so you will not have the temptation to run out of the house in the morning without your lunch.
- Healthy snacks: pack a small low-fat yogurt, a pair of whole wheat crackers with peanut butter, or vegetables with hummus.

Myth: Eating healthy foods is too expensive.

Truth: Eating better does not have to cost a lot of money. Many people think that fresh foods are healthier than canned or frozen foods. For example, some people think that spinach is better raw than frozen or canned. However, some canned or frozen fruits and vegetables provide as many nutrients as fresh ones and at a lower cost. Choose canned vegetables low in salt and canned fruits in their own juice or in water. Do not forget to rinse canned vegetables to remove excess salt.Some canned seafood, such as tuna, is healthy, inexpensive and easy to keep in the dispensation.Other healthy sources of protein that do not cost much are lentils, peas or canned beans, frozen or packaged in sheath.

Tip: Look at the nutritional information on canned, frozen and wrapped foods. Look for foods that are rich in calcium, fiber, potassium, protein and vitamin D. Also look for foods that are low in added sugars, saturated fats and sodium.

Myth: Physical activity only counts if I can do it for long periods of time.

Truth: You do not need to do physical activity for long periods to achieve your 2½ to 5 hours of activity each week. Experts advise doing aerobic activity for periods of 10 minutes or more at a time.You can distribute these sessions throughout the week.

Tip: Plan to do at least 10 minutes of physical activity three times a day for 5 or more days a week. This will help you reach the 2½ hour goal. Take a few minutes of your work to take a walk. Use the stairs Get off the bus one stop before yours.Go dancing with your friends. It does not matter whether they are short or long periods, these periods of activity can add up to the total amount of physical activity you need each week.

Myth: Eating meat is bad for my health and makes it harder for me to lose weight.

Truth: Eating small amounts of lean meat (the one with little fat) can be part of a healthy plan to lose weight. While it is true that chicken, fish, pork and red meat contain a little cholesterol and saturated fat, they also contain healthy nutrients such as iron, protein and zinc.

Tip: Select the cuts of meat that have less fat and remove all the fat you see. The cuts of meat with less fat include chicken breast ("chicken breast"), pork loin ("pork loin"), beef steak ("beef round steak") and extra lean ground beef ("extra lean ground beef"). You should also look at the size of the portions.Try to eat meat or chicken in 3-ounce servings (about 8.5 grams) or less.

Myth: Milk and milk products make me fat and unhealthy.

Truth: Fat-free or low-fat cheese, milk and yogurt are as nutritious as products made with whole milk, but have less fat and calories. Milk products, also known as dairy products, have protein that serves to increase muscle mass and to help organs work well. They also have calcium that serves to strengthen bones. Most milks and some yogurts are enriched with vitamin D that helps the body use calcium.Most people who live in the United States do not get enough calcium or vitamin D. Milk products are an easy way to get more of these nutrients.

Tip: You should try to consume 3 cups per day of non-fat or low-fat milk or its equivalent in milk products. This may include soy-based drinks enriched with vitamins. If you can not digest lactose (the type of sugar found in milk products), choose milk products that do not contain lactose or have low levels of lactose. You can also choose other foods and drinks that contain calcium and vitamin D, such as:

- Calcium: canned salmon, dark green leafy vegetables such as cabbage or kale, and soy-based drinks or tofu made with calcium sulfate.
- Vitamin D: cereals or soy-based drinks.

Myth: Being a vegetarian will help me lose weight and be healthier.

Truth: Studies show that people who follow a vegetarian eating plan usually consume fewer calories and fats than people who are not vegetarians. Some studies have also found that vegetarian-style eating is associated with a lower level of obesity, blood pressure and risk of heart disease. Vegetarians also have less body fat than people who are not vegetarians.However, both vegetarians and non-vegetarians can choose foods that are not so healthy that they can affect their weight by making them go up. For example, they may eat large quantities of high-fat, low-calorie foods with little nutritional value

Tip: If you decide to follow a vegetarian diet plan, be sure to ingest the nutrients you normally get from animal products like cheeses, eggs, meat and milk. In the table below, you will find a list of the nutrients that may be missing in a vegetarian diet with some foods and drinks that may help you meet your needs for those nutrients.

CHAPTER FOUR:
Exersice For Endomorph

The endomorph must choose a type of training to strengthen its metabolism. The training must have circuits, super series, short breaks, etc, all these are beneficial in their purpose of building a muscular and defined physique. In your training it is recommended to use between 12 and 15 repetitions, short breaks (30 to 60 seconds).

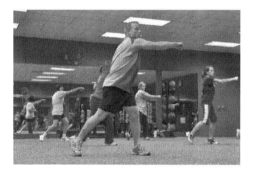

Cardio: Obviously a need for every athlete who practices weights either in volume or cut and much more important for an endomorph.

Weekly work with weights for endomorphs: 5 days, between 5 and 7 hours

At first, you will progress very little respect to the weights, but in the second month, you will start to progress faster.

Always paying special attention to make the correct technique in your exercises.

In training, you have to alternate between heavy training of high-intensity training with more repetitions and volume.

FULLBODY BASIC ROUTINE FOR ENDOMORPHOS

Monday

- Bench press: 4 × 15
- Push-ups: 4 × 15
- Curl bar: 4 × 12
- Curl hammer: 4 × 12
- Femoral lying down: 4 × 15
- Squat: 4 × 20

Tuesday

- Dominant: 4 × 15
- Rowing dumbbells: 4 × 12
- Military
- press: 4 × 15 Lateral lifts: 4 × 15
- Triceps funds: 4 × 15
- French press: 4 × 15

Thursday

- Press inclined bench: 4 × 15
- Pectoral bottoms: 4 × 15
- Curl bar: 4 × 12
- Hammer curl: 4 × 12
- Strides: 4 × 15
- Twins: 4 × 15

Friday

- Dominated narrow grip: 4 × 15
- Pulley at chest: 4 × 15
- Lateral elevations: 4 × 15
- Bird: 4 × 15
- French press
- press: 4 × 12 Pulley: 4 × 12

ADVANCED ROUTINE ENDOMORPHOS (5 DAYS)

Monday: Back and twins

- Pulley pulley to the front: heating 2 x 20 + 12 - 10 - 8 - 6 - 6 - 5 rep.
- Rest between sets of this exercise 2 minutes approximately.
- Triserie: Rowing with bar 4 series x 10 - 6 repetitions
- Rowing in low pulley 4 series x 10 - 8 repetitions
- Pulling rigid arms 4 series x 15 - 12 repetitions
- Rest between these three exercises, none, at the end of the trilogy, between

- 1.5 and 2 minutes.
- Superset: Twin - soleo sitting 4 x 12
- Twin donkey 4 x 12 - 15

Tuesday: Chest and abdomen

- Bench press: heating 3 x 20 + 12 - 10 - 8 - 6 - 6 - 5 rep.
- Triserie: Upper press with dumbbells 4 x 10 - 6
- Openings 4 x 10 - 8
- Contractor 4 x 15 - 12
- Superset: Shrugs for upper abdomen 4 x maximas
- Lower abdomen 4 x maximas

Wednesday: Arms

- Curl with bar: heating 2 x 20 + 12 - 10 - 8 - 6 - 6 rep.
- Superset: Curl Scott 4 x 10 - 6
- Alternate curl inclined 4 x 15 - 12
- French Press: heating 2 x 20 + 12 - 10 - 8 - 6 - 6 rep.
- Superset: Triceps pulley 4 x 10 - 6
- Triceps bar Z sitting 4 x 15 - 12

Thursday: Legs

- Squat: heating 2 x 20 + 12 - 10 - 8 - 6 - 6 - 5 rep.
- Giant series: Inclined press 4 x 10 - 6
- Squat Jack 4 x 10 - 8
- Extensions machine 4 x 15 - 12
- Femoral curl 4 x 12 - 10

Friday: Shoulders and forearms (optional)

- Military press: heating 2 x 20 + 12 - 10 - 8 - 6 - 6 - 5
- Triserie: Rowing stand with bar 4 x 10 - 6
- Lateral lifts 4 x 12 - 10
- Bird 4 x 12 - 10
- If you decide to work the forearms:
- Superset: Flexors 4 x 15 - 12
- Extenders 4 x 15 – 12

CHAPTER FIVE:
The Best Weight Loss Supplements For Endomorph

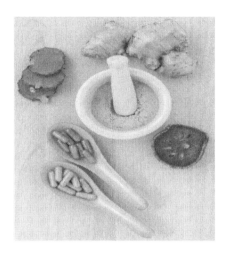

Some of the best weight loss supplements are made from the most natural of ingredients. These ingredients help an individual lose unwanted fat through a in the body coupled with a metabolic boost. Natural ingredients which stimulate thermogenesis in the body are substances like apple cider vinegar, ginseng, green tea, cinnamon, and cayenne pepper.These supplements are likely to "rev up" the metabolism, tell the body to use fat storage for energy and ultimately induce thermogenesis. Best of all, these top weight loss supplements may be exactly what a person needs in conjunction with diet and exercise to change their life and quickly lose unwanted fat. All around the world, and especially in developed countries, obesity seems to be to almost epidemic proportions. Living in a fast paced world and a 24 hour society, it's easy to eat fast foods, sugary snacks and takeaways. Never before have our diets been so bad and this is having an adverse affect on our health and confidence.

If you are struggling with your weight and you want a way out help is at hand if you find the best weight loss supplement that is right for you. The difficult part will be figuring out which one will work for you. Weight loss supplements come in several different forms.These supplements can suppress your appetite, block carbohydrates, boost your energy, promote balance in your thyroid and block fats.

The weight loss pill that will be best for you will depend on the reasons why you are overweight. For example, if you have a thyroid problem, you may want to take a supplement that will help to allow your thyroid to work properly. If you have a difficult time saying no to extra portions or snacking, an appetite suppressant could give you the help that you need.

Some of the most popular weight loss supplements include Hoodia, green tea extract and caralluma fimbriate. Each of these are derived from a natural source and they each serve a different function. Hoodia and Caralluma helps to control your appetite and green tea extract increases your metabolism.A combination of these may end up being just what you need in order to lose weight.Of course, the best weight loss supplement will vary from individual to individual. There are plenty out there, however, that will provide your body with what it needs in order to strike a balance. Look for a product that contains all of these various supplements or a combination that works best for you.

Best Supplements for Endomorphs

Aside from the proper diet and exercise, it is also necessary for you to learn more about the best supplements for endomorphs. Ensure that you take them regularly to increase your chances of maintaining a healthy weight. Whey protein – One supplement that works well for endomorphs is whey protein. It is a good choice as it is nutritionally complete. This means that it can provide your diet with the protein-building blocks and amino acids your daily meal plan needs.

As an endomorph, it is greatly possible that you are carefully monitoring your nutrient intake as a means of preventing unwanted weight gain. In this case, whey protein can help.It has a predetermined serving size as well as protein content, which promotes further ease when it comes to monitoring your protein consumption every day.What is even better about it is that it is now available in various flavors. With that, you can add variety to your daily diet, which is a good thing, especially if you are still on the stage of restricting calories.

BCAA – Branched-chain amino acids (BCAAs) are also among the most vital supplements that an endomorph should take.It would be best to take this supplement during and right after you work out.It is because this supplement can aid in effective muscle recovery and endurance.

Note that your workout plans will most likely focus on intense intervals and big movements. This is the main reason why you need to have the proper fuel so you can put more effort during your training.You can get such fuel by supplementing with BCAA.

Fat-burning supplements – It is also advisable to take supplements that improve the ability of your body to burn fats.In this case, you can take certain herbal supplements, minerals, or vitamins that are proven scientifically to stimulate weight loss.

Keys About Fat Burners

What's good about most fat burners today, is that they can not only speed up the ability of your body to burn fat, they also provide a boost in energy to help you power through workouts. They are also helpful in reducing your appetite and increasing your metabolism.

Myths And Facts About Weight Loss Supplements
Due to the many weight loss supplements available in the market, there are many myths that surround them. Here are some of the myths:

You don't need to exercise or diet if you are taking the supplements

Many people tend to think that they don't need to exercise or diet when they are taking weight loss supplements. The truth is that you need to exercise and diet when taking the supplements. The best diet that you should take is a low-fat diet. According to experts, you should ensure that your meal contains no more than 15 grams of fat.

When it comes to exercises, you should engage in both cardio and muscle building exercises.To be on the safe side, you should exercise at least 30 minutes daily. If you can't exercise daily, you should exercise at least three times a week.

If it's on the store shelf, it's safe

Many people tend to believe that the weight loss supplements on the store shelves are FDA approved.You should note that FDA approves just a small number of supplements; therefore, there is no guarantee that the medications are safe for you.To ensure that the medications are safe, you need to research them.One of the best places to research is online. Here you need to visit the various review sites and see what different people have to say about the products. As always you should avoid a product with many negative reviews.

Natural weight loss supplements don't have any side effects

While many manufacturers say that natural supplements don't have any side effects, you should be cautious of the supplements.This is because according to experts, anything that causes an effect can cause a side effect. This means that you should be very careful when taking the supplements. To ensure that you are safe you should always contact your doctor before taking the supplements.

Bitter orange is a safe substitute for ephedra

While bitter orange contains synephrine which is similar to ephedra, ephedra is not safe. This is because it has been shown to bring about increased blood pressure and arrhythmias. In fact it was banned in 2004 by FDA for bringing about a number of high profile deaths.These are some of the myths surrounding the various weight loss supplements.While there are some supplements that are safe for consumption, there are others that are not safe.To be on the safe side always consult your doctor before taking any supplements.

CHAPTER SIX:
How To Improve Your Eating Habits

When it comes to eating, we all have deep-rooted habits. Some are good ("I always have my breakfast") and others are not so good ("I always leave the plate clean"). Although many eating habits acquired from childhood does not mean it is too late to change them. Sudden and radical changes in eating habits, such as not eating more than cabbage soup, can lead to short-term weight loss. But these exaggerated changes are not healthy or good and will not help in the long term. To improve eating habits permanently, you need an approach that Reflects, Substitute and Reinforces.

- REFLECT on all your eating habits, both good and bad, as well as the things that trigger you to eat unhealthily.
- REPLACE your unhealthy eating habits with healthier ones.
- REINFORCE their new eating habits.

Reflect, replace and reinforce: A process to improve your eating habits

1. Make a list of your eating habits. Keeping a "food diary" for a few days where you write down everything you eat and

the time you do it will help you discover your habits. For example, you may realize that you always want something sweet when you feel low energy in the afternoon. Use menu planning to compile the list. It is good to write down how you felt when you decided to eat, especially if you were not hungry. Was I tired or stressed?

2. Underline the habits on the list that are causing you to eat more than necessary. Eating habits that can often lead to weight gain are:

- Eat very fast
- Eat everything that is served on the plate
- Eat when you are not hungry
- Eat standing (you can make it eat without thinking about what you eat or very fast)
- Always eat dessert
- Skip meals (or just breakfast)

3. Review the unhealthy eating habits you have underlined. Be sure to identify all the factors that trigger those habits. Identify some of the ones you will try to change first. Do not stop congratulating yourself on the things you do well.Maybe you almost always eat fruit for dessert or drink low-fat or defatted milk. These are good habits! By recognizing your accomplishments you will feel motivated to make more changes.

4. Make a list of "triggers" by reviewing your food diary will be more aware of where and when "trigger" factors arise to eat without being hungry. Write down how you usually feel

on those occasions.Often an environmental "trigger" or a particular mood is what drives us to eat without being hungry. Common triggers that drive people to eat when they are not hungry:

- Open a drawer and find your favorite snack.
- Sit at home to watch TV.
- Before or after a meeting or a stressful situation at work.
- Get home from work and have no idea what you are going to eat.
- Have someone offer you a dish that he made "just for you"!
- Pass in front of a sweet dish on a counter.
- Sit in the workroom near the vending machine for treats or snacks.
- See a plate of donuts in the morning during a work meeting.
- Spend all the mornings at the window of your favorite fast food restaurant.
- Feeling bored or tired and thinking that eating something will boost your spirits.

5. Circle the "triggers" of the list you face on a daily or weekly basis. Gathering with your family on Thanksgiving Day can be a "trigger" factor for overeating.It would be good to have a plan ready to counteract these factors.But for now, focus on the ones you have most often.

6. Ask yourself the following for each "trigger" factor that you marked in a circle:

- Is there anything I can do to avoid this trigger or this situation? This option works best with some triggers that are independent of others. For example, could you take a different path to work to avoid stopping at your favorite fast food restaurant? Is there another place in the workroom where you can sit that is not near the vending machine?
- Of the things that I can not avoid, can I do something different that is healthier? Obviously, you can not avoid all situations that trigger unhealthy eating habits, such as work meetings. In these circumstances, evaluate your options. Could you suggest or bring healthy snacks and drinks? Could you offer to take notes to distract your attention from those refreshments? Could you sit further away from the food so that it is not easy for you to grab something? Could I eat a healthy snack before the meeting?

7. Replace unhealthy habits with new healthy habits. For example: when reflecting on your eating habits, you may realize that you eat too fast when you are alone. To counter this, agree to have lunch every week with a co-worker or invite a neighbor to dinner one night a week. Other strategies may be placing the cutlery on the plate between bites or minimizing other distractions (such as watching the news at dinner) with which we can not pay attention to the time it takes to eat or the amount of food.

Here are more ideas to replace unhealthy habits:

- Eat more slowly. If you eat very quickly, you may end up with all the food on the plate without realizing that it has already been filled.
- Eat only when you really are hungry, instead of eating because you are tired, anguished or with any other mood. If you realize that you are not eating hungry but because you feel bored or distressed, start doing something else that does not involve eating. You may feel better with a quick walk or by calling a friend.
- Plan meals ahead of time to make sure they will be healthy and well-balanced.

8. Reinforce your new healthy habits and be patient with yourself. Habits are formed over time, they are not adopted overnight. When you see that you are practicing a habit that is unhealthy, quickly stop and ask yourself: Why am I doing this? When did I start doing it? What do I need to change? Do not be too hard on yourself or think that a mistake will ruin a day of healthy habits. You can achieve it! You can do it one day at a time!

CONCLUSION

Even if you are prone to gaining weight, there is still hope for you if you have an endomorph body type. What you have to do is to learn about the ideal diet plan for you, stick to the right exercise regimen, and take the necessary supplements. You will notice that you are shedding off pounds in no time if you strictly stick to a healthy lifestyle and the best endomorph diet and exercise plan. Losing weight can seem like an uphill battle when your efforts don't pay off. Understanding your individual body type, as well as the unique challenges faced by endomorphs, may help you drop pounds and hit your fitness goals. Maintain a low intake of refined carbs, get plenty of regular physical activity, and practice portion control. These are all healthy behaviors recommended for most people.Sticking with this routine may help you shed excess pounds — and keep the weight off. Endomorphs carry more body fat than other types and tend to be softer and curvier.While this may sound like a disadvantage, they can lose fat with correct eating habits and by training hard, they can afford to lose a small amount of muscle on the way.In fact many of the best fitness models are endomorphs with a little mesomorph and when trained can have a curvy shapely toned body.

If you've found this book helpful in any way, a review on Amazon is very much appreciated and if you liked it you might also like:

"The Mediterranean Diet: (2 Books in 1) Mediterranean Diet for Beginners + Mediterranean Diet Plan" by Emma Moore

"Alkaline Diet for Beginners: A Scientifically Based Guide and Cookbook to Eat Well and Heal the Electric Body featuring Easy Recipes for Energy Reset and Weight Loss" by Emma Moore

Made in the USA
Middletown, DE
28 July 2021